# How to Succeed on Nursing Placements

Sara Miller McCune founded SAGE Publishing in 1965 to support the dissemination of usable knowledge and educate a global community. SAGE publishes more than 1000 journals and over 800 new books each year, spanning a wide range of subject areas. Our growing selection of library products includes archives, data, case studies and video. SAGE remains majority owned by our founder and after her lifetime will become owned by a charitable trust that secures the company's continued independence.

Los Angeles | London | New Delhi | Singapore | Washington DC | Melbourne

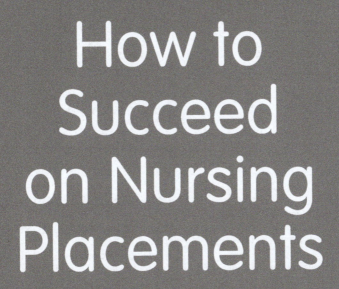

# How to Succeed on Nursing Placements

Karen Elcock

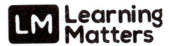

LM Learning Matters

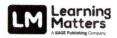

Learning Matters
A SAGE Publishing Company
1 Oliver's Yard
55 City Road
London EC1Y 1SP

SAGE Publications Inc.
2455 Teller Road
Thousand Oaks, California 91320

SAGE Publications India Pvt Ltd
B 1/I 1 Mohan Cooperative Industrial Area
Mathura Road
New Delhi 110 044

SAGE Publications Asia-Pacific Pte Ltd
3 Church Street
#10-04 Samsung Hub
Singapore 049483

Editor: Laura Walmsley
Development editor: Sarah Turpie
Senior project editor: Chris Marke
Project management: Swales & Willis Ltd, Exeter, Devon
Marketing manager: Camille Richmond
Cover design: Wendy Scott
Typeset by: C&M Digitals (P) Ltd, Chennai, India
Printed in the UK

**Library of Congress Control Number: 2019953483**

**British Library Cataloguing in Publication Data**

A catalogue record for this book is available from the British Library

ISBN 978-1-5264-6997-7
ISBN 978-1-5264-6996-0 (pbk)

# Contents

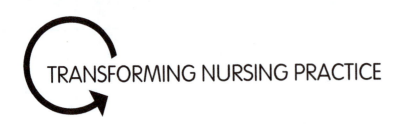

# TRANSFORMING NURSING PRACTICE

*Transforming Nursing Practice* is a series tailor made for pre-registration students nurses. Each book in the series is:

 Affordable

 Full of active learning features

 Mapped to the NMC Standards of proficiency for registered nurses

 Focused on applying theory to practice

Each book addresses a core topic and they have been carefully developed to be simple to use, quick to read and written in clear language.

An invaluable series of books that explicitly relates to the NMC standards. Each book covers a different topic that students need to explore in order to develop into a qualified nurse... I would recommend this series to all Pre-Registered nursing students whatever their field or year of study.

**LINDA ROBSON,**
Senior Lecturer at Edge Hill University

Many titles in the series are on our recommended reading list and for good reason - the content is up to date and easy to read. These are the books that actually get used beyond training and into your nursing career.

**EMMA LYDON,**
Adult Student Nursing

## ABOUT THE SERIES EDITORS

**DR MOOI STANDING** is an Independent Academic Nursing Consultant (UK and international) responsible for the core knowledge, personal and professional learning skills titles. She has invaluable experience as an NMC Quality Assurance Reviewer of educational programmes, and as a Professional Regulator Panellist on the NMC Practice Committee. Mooi is also a Board member of Special Olympics Malaysia.

**DR SANDRA WALKER** is a Clinical Academic in Mental Health working between North Bristol Trust and Southern Health Trust. She is series editor for the mental health nursing titles. She is a Qualified Mental Health Nurse with a wide range of clinical experience spanning 30 years and spent several years working as a mental health lecturer at Southampton University.

# BESTSELLING TEXTBOOKS

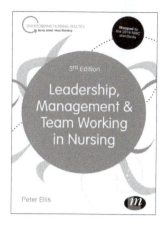

3rd Edition

Leadership, Management & Team Working in Nursing

Peter Ellis

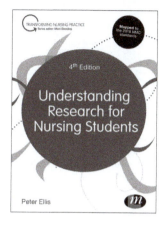

4th Edition

Understanding Research for Nursing Students

Peter Ellis

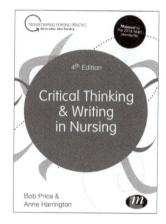

4th Edition

Critical Thinking & Writing in Nursing

Bob Price & Anne Harrington

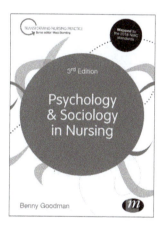

3rd Edition

Psychology & Sociology in Nursing

Benny Goodman

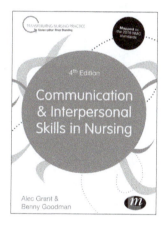

4th Edition

Communication & Interpersonal Skills in Nursing

Alec Grant & Benny Goodman

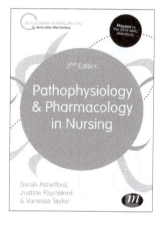

2nd Edition

Pathophysiology & Pharmacology in Nursing

Sarah Ashelford, Justine Raynsford & Vanessa Taylor

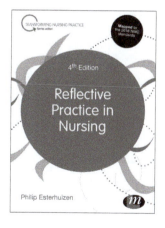

4th Edition

Reflective Practice in Nursing

Philip Esterhuizen

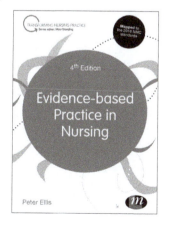

4th Edition

Evidence-based Practice in Nursing

Peter Ellis

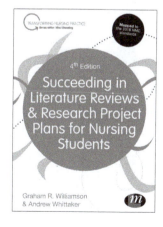

4th Edition

Succeeding in Literature Reviews & Research Project Plans for Nursing Students

Graham R. Williamson & Andrew Whittaker

You can find a full list of textbooks in the
*Transforming Nursing Practice* series at
https://uk.sagepub.com

# About the authors

**Karen Elcock** is Head of Programmes – Pre-Registration Nursing and Deputy Head of School at Kingston University and St George's, University of London. By background an adult critical care nurse, she has worked in nurse education for 30 years. Her passion is the student experience in practice and developing staff who support students on placement. She is a prolific writer of books and articles on pre-registration nursing and education in practice.

**Karen Chandler** is Associate Professor and Director of Practice in the School of Nursing at Kingston University and St George's, University of London. Her background is neonatal and paediatric critical care, and she continues to work clinically in paediatric and adult emergency care. She is passionate about student support in clinical practice and is undertaking doctoral studies examining conceptual issues of fitness to practise in nurse education.

**Jane Dundas** is Senior Lecturer in Clinical Leadership and Management at Kingston University and St George's, University of London. She ran her own business for many years before returning to nursing as clinical nursing lead for stroke services in acute and community settings. Using these experiences, Jane enables nurses and healthcare professionals to improve the quality of care for patients. Jane has published chapters in books as well as in journals and conference papers.

**Martyn Keen** is Senior Lecturer in Mental Health Nursing at Kingston University and St George's, University of London. He has over 28 years' experience in mental healthcare, specialising clinically in adult mental health community care and early intervention services. He is also an experienced educator, working with multi-professional students across undergraduate and postgraduate programmes as well as workforce development. Martyn's passion lies in student health and well-being and developing innovative learning approaches.

**Sonia Levett** lives in Sydney, Australia, and has been a registered nurse for 30 years. She specialises in the post-anaesthetic care unit and has worked as a clinical nurse specialist. She has a passion for education, imparting her experience as well as supporting and empowering nurses to reach their potential. She has acted as a clinical facilitator for undergraduates and a nurse educator for new graduates. She currently works at Macquarie University Hospital.

**Michelle McBride** is Senior Lecturer in Nurse Education at Roehampton University, London (previously at Kingston University). By background a district nurse, she has worked in nurse education for six years. Her passion is to ensure all students have a community focus throughout their training, with a particular emphasis on experiences outside the standard curriculum. She has published articles relating to wound care and learning through simulation.

**Kath Sharples** is Nurse Manager, Education and Research at Macquarie University Hospital, Sydney, Australia. As a specialist nurse educator, her expertise is in work-based professional development and operational/strategic education leadership across private and public healthcare organisations, higher education providers and aged care. She has international experience in the strategic planning and delivery of innovative approaches to continuing professional development and the translation of evaluative research into evidence-based best practice.

**Robert Stanley** is Senior Lecturer in Learning Disability Nursing at Kingston University and St George's, University of London. He has worked in nurse education for 20 years and is the academic lead for supporting students with additional needs. His approach to teaching and learning is that all students' entitlement to access and participate in a course is anticipated, acknowledged and taken into account.

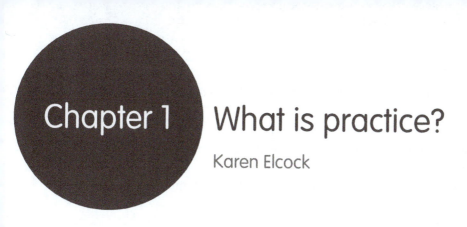

# Chapter 1  What is practice?

Karen Elcock

---

## NMC Standards of Proficiency for Registered Nurses

This chapter will address the following platforms and proficiencies:

**Platform 1: Being an accountable professional**

Registered nurses act in the best interests of people, putting them first and providing nursing care that is person-centred, safe and compassionate. They act professionally at all times and use their knowledge and experience to make evidence-based decisions about care. They communicate effectively, are role models for others, and are accountable for their actions. Registered nurses continually reflect on their practice and keep abreast of new and emerging developments in nursing, health and care.

At the point of registration, the registered nurse will be able to:

1.1 understand and act in accordance with *The Code: Professional Standards of Practice and Behaviour for Nurses, Midwives and Nursing Associates*, and fulfil all registration requirements.

1.2 understand and apply relevant legal, regulatory and governance requirements, policies, and ethical frameworks, including any mandatory reporting duties, to all areas of practice, differentiating where appropriate between the devolved legislatures of the United Kingdom.

1.13 demonstrate the skills and abilities required to develop, manage and maintain appropriate relationships with people, their families, carers and colleagues.

---

## Chapter aims

After reading this chapter, you will be able to:

- appreciate why practice is an essential part of your programme;

*(Continued)*

(Continued)

- demonstrate an understanding of the regulatory requirements that govern your learning in practice;
- identify the key policies that are essential for safe practice;
- appreciate how skills and simulated learning are an important component of practice; and
- consider the differing expectations of the university and placement providers when you attend practice.

# Introduction

There is little doubt that practice is, for most students, the 'best part' of their course. It makes up at least 50 per cent of a pre-registration nursing programme, which demonstrates its importance in preparing you to become a registered nurse. It is this balance between theory and practice that makes a nursing course very attractive to many students. It offers the opportunity to apply the theory learnt in university to the real world of practice and also bring the learning from practice back to university to inform class seminars, discussions and assignments. One of the challenges with learning in practice is that it is inevitably very messy and unpredictable. At university, you will have a timetable with scheduled classes that will develop your knowledge incrementally across the programme. Practice is far less predictable, and you will come across things you have not yet learnt at university. This will require you to undertake additional research and reading alongside your course activities to help you make sense of what you see. In addition, you will be faced with situations that will challenge you both emotionally and intellectually as well as situations that will provide you with memories that will stay with you forever. However, you will not make this journey alone, and there will always be support available to you both in practice and at university from a range of staff. We will look at these people later in the book.

This chapter sets the scene for many of the chapters later in this book. It looks at why practice (both out on placement and in the clinical skills laboratory) is such an important part of your programme. Practice is essential in developing the skills and knowledge you need to meet the requirements set by the Nursing and Midwifery Council (NMC) and so register as a nurse at the end of your programme. Much of the way learning in practice is organised and structured is governed by the NMC education and programme standards (NMC, 2018b, 2018c, 2018d), and so we will look at their requirements to help you understand why your university has some rules and regulations around practice that are non-negotiable. The NMC exists to protect the public, and so in addition to their standards, which inform the development of your programme, there are also a number of additional standards, guidelines and policies published by them to ensure safe practice and also to ensure you stay within the law. Some of these are key for practice, so we will explore them, why they are important and what they mean for your practice. We will end the chapter by considering the expectations of both the university and **practice partners**, who provide your placements during your course.

# What do we mean by practice?

Practice relates to both the placements that you will be allocated to and to the learning that takes place in **skills and simulation suites or laboratories** (often called skills labs). Placements are provided by practice learning partners, who have a joint responsibility with the university to ensure the quality of your programme.

## Activity 1.1   Evidence-based practice

You may have selected your university based on where you will have an opportunity to undertake your placements, or you may not have considered this as important as the university itself.

Do you know who all the practice partners at your university are that will be providing placements for you, and so where you may potentially be allocated to? If you are unsure, check the university website or the information on practice placements your university has provided you with.

*As this activity is based on your own observation, there is no outline answer at the end of the chapter.*

Depending on your reasons for choosing your university and the research you undertook to find out about the placement partners it works with, Activity 1.1 may or may not have provided some surprises for you. Regardless, the types of placements you will gain experience in are varied. They include hospitals, community and primary care trusts, GP practices, the independent, charity and voluntary sectors, **integrated health and social care** settings, schools and colleges, and nursing and residential care homes (RCN, 2017a). Both placements and skills and simulation suites provide students with a range of practice learning opportunities that are designed to:

> *allow students to develop and meet the* Standards of proficiency for registered nurses *to deliver safe and effective care to a diverse range of people across the four fields of nursing practice.*
>
> (NMC, 2018d, p10)

Practice provides you with the opportunity to learn the skills that will be essential to you as you progress on your course and in your career as a nurse. However, it is not just about learning practical skills; practice also offers you the opportunity to apply the theory learnt in university to the real world of practice and develop your professional identity as a nurse. The importance of placements to students is described by Jenni Middleton, the editor of *Nursing Times,* when she says:

*Students tell us over and over again that their placement is one of the most important aspects of their training. A positive placement experience will not only teach good practice but will also coach students in how to develop relationships with their peers and patients.*

(J. Middleton, 2017)

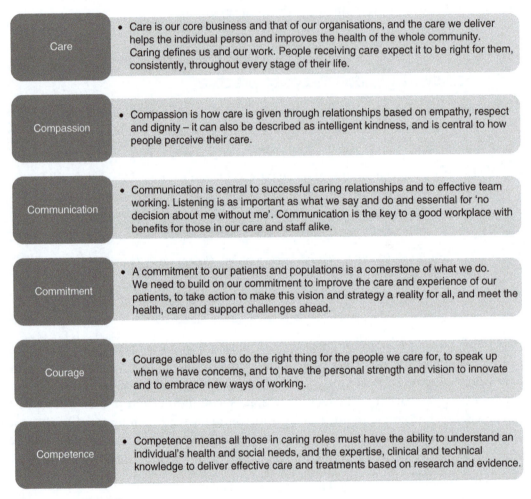

**Care**
- Care is our core business and that of our organisations, and the care we deliver helps the individual person and improves the health of the whole community. Caring defines us and our work. People receiving care expect it to be right for them, consistently, throughout every stage of their life.

**Compassion**
- Compassion is how care is given through relationships based on empathy, respect and dignity – it can also be described as intelligent kindness, and is central to how people perceive their care.

**Communication**
- Communication is central to successful caring relationships and to effective team working. Listening is as important as what we say and do and essential for 'no decision about me without me'. Communication is the key to a good workplace with benefits for those in our care and staff alike.

**Commitment**
- A commitment to our patients and populations is a cornerstone of what we do. We need to build on our commitment to improve the care and experience of our patients, to take action to make this vision and strategy a reality for all, and meet the health, care and support challenges ahead.

**Courage**
- Courage enables us to do the right thing for the people we care for, to speak up when we have concerns, and to have the personal strength and vision to innovate and to embrace new ways of working.

**Competence**
- Competence means all those in caring roles must have the ability to understand an individual's health and social needs, and the expertise, clinical and technical knowledge to deliver effective care and treatments based on research and evidence.

*Figure 1.1*  The 6Cs

*Source*: Department of Health and NHS Commissioning Board (2012). Reproduced with permission under the Open Government Licence

Developing (professional) relationships with your peers (students and other registered healthcare professionals) and patients and their carers is important in developing your professional identity. These relationships form part of the **professional socialisation** process of learning the skills, attitudes, values and behaviours required to become a nurse (Maginnis, 2018). Role models, particularly in practice, are highly influential in the development of the professional traits required in students. During your time in practice and in university, you will not only learn the skills and knowledge required, but more importantly acquire and develop the professional values and behaviours required of a nurse.

In 2012, *Compassion in Practice* was published, which identified six values and behaviours that are seen as fundamental to, and should underpin, all care wherever it takes place. These six values and behaviours have become known as the 6Cs (Department of Health and NHS Commissioning Board, 2012) and are shown in Figure 1.1. You will find the 6Cs are a significant part of your nursing curriculum, be it in class, in the skills lab or within your Practice Assessment Document, as there is an expectation that they underpin everything you do as a nurse.

# The role of skills and simulation in practice learning

Skills and simulation are an important part of your practice learning. These may be delivered in blocks or as a regular event on a defined day each week. Either way, you will find they run throughout the length of your programme.

The NMC defines simulation as:

> *An artificial representation of a real world practice scenario that supports student development through experiential learning with the opportunity for repetition, feedback, evaluation and reflection. Effective simulation facilitates safety by enhancing knowledge, behaviours and skills.*

> (NMC, 2018d, p18)

While the NMC describes it as an artificial representation, the technology that is now available means that the simulations can feel very real. For example, high-fidelity simulations use computerised mannequins that can be programmed to demonstrate a wide range of patient conditions and clinical signs, which can change depending on how you respond to their needs. It is not just about technology, however; many universities now use role players who play the part of a patient, service user, carer or child within a defined scenario. Role players offer students a more realistic element to their learning, and in particular a more genuine experience of what it is like to communicate with the individual. After the simulation, the student can receive honest feedback on what it was like for the role player in being cared for by the student and the quality of the student's communication and demonstration of empathy and compassion. You will find your university uses a wide range of approaches to simulation; Table 1.1 lists some you may come across.

| Low-fidelity simulation | Paper or computer-based tasks, basic mannequins, task trainers (e.g. an arm for cannulation). |
|---|---|
| High-fidelity simulation | Computerised mannequins that can mimic changes in clinical parameters and provide responses/feedback to interventions by the student. |
| Standardised patients or simulated patients | Role players who portray patients, carers, hospital staff (particularly good for interpersonal and communication skills). |
| Serious gaming | Use of computer-based games for the purpose of education as opposed to fun. |
| Virtual worlds | Run on desktop computers. |
| Virtual reality | Computer-generated worlds, both visual and auditory. |

*Table 1.1*   Types of simulation

Simulation is used to prepare students for clinical practice – for example, teaching core clinical nursing skills such as handwashing, taking clinical observations (pulse, respiratory rate, blood pressure), moving and handling, or basic cardiopulmonary resuscitation (CPR), as well as offering students an opportunity to practise skills that may not be easily available when out on placement. Simulation also offers opportunities to apply some of the skills you have seen or used in practice to new scenarios and polish your skills further. However, it is not just about practical clinical skills. Simulation, especially with role players acting as patients, carers or healthcare workers, can provide you with the opportunity to develop your communication and **therapeutic skills**, starting with relatively simple skills such as patient assessment to highly complex scenarios such as **conflict management**, responding to people with **mental distress**, and **clinical decision-making**. As well as using simulation to help students develop their skills, many universities use **Objective Structured Clinical Assessments or Examinations (OSCAs or OSCEs)** in the skills labs to assess student competence in both clinical and interpersonal skills. Skills and simulation therefore offer a wide range of benefits, including:

- opportunities to rehearse skills prior to entering practice;
- statutory and mandatory training in core skills required in practice;
- mistakes can be made in safety before being discussed and corrected;
- students are provided with an opportunity to practise skills that are less commonly seen in practice or that are more difficult to achieve;
- simulations can be set up at differing levels of complexity depending on the student's competence level or stage in the programme;
- immediate feedback can be provided verbally or by the student reviewing videos of the simulation;
- opportunities to undertake simulations with other health and social care professionals;

- involvement of service users in the development of scenarios or as role players to enhance reality; and
- opportunities to reflect on performance with academic staff and peers.

The opportunity to reflect on your performance is an essential part of the simulation experience and is part of the debriefing process. This may take place during or after the simulation exercise, on a one-to-one basis or with peers. Academic staff may use video recordings of your performance to help you critically reflect on your performance, consider your feelings in the simulation and your responses to what was taking place, and identify areas of strength and areas for further development. Simulation is an important part of your pre-registration programme, and one that your university will take seriously, as the case study below about Rosa shows. Read the case study and then consider Activity 1.2.

## Case study: Rosa

Rosa is a first-year student who has turned up for her first skills lesson at university. The information provided before the session said that students must follow the dress code policy, so she has put her hair up and removed her jewellery. However, she has only had new acrylic nails applied at the weekend, so she decides not to remove them. When she enters the skills lab, the lecturer is checking that each student is appropriately dressed, and when she sees Rosa's nails she tells her she that she will need to remove them before she can participate in class. Rosa argues that the skills lab is not real, and she does not understand why she should remove them.

## Activity 1.2   Critical thinking

Why do you think the university requires students to adhere to the dress code when in skills and simulation labs?

*An outline answer to this activity is given at the end of the chapter.*

Your university will have rules regarding your appearance, behaviour and timekeeping when out in practice as well as when attending simulation events. The next section will look at some of these expectations and some additional NMC requirements specific to practice.

# Regulatory requirements for practice

The NMC makes a number of stipulations concerning practice learning (Figure 1.2). Your university has to ensure these requirements are met during your programme, and this will have been checked by the NMC when your programme was developed. The NMC will also check that the university has systems and processes in place to ensure students meet these requirements when they make any monitoring visits in the future.

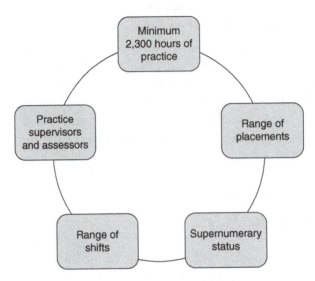

*Figure 1.2*  NMC requirements for practice

*Source*: NMC (2018d)

Over the length of your course, you are required to complete a minimum of 2,300 hours, experience the full range of hours (shifts) that nurses work, have a range of different experiences in clinical practice that allow you to meet the NMC proficiencies, and be supernumerary when on placement. Let us look at each of these in more detail.

## Practice hours

The number of hours you must complete is determined by standards that have been agreed by the European Union (EU). The *EU Directive 2005/36/EC of the European Parliament and of the Council on the Recognition of Professional Qualifications* was devised to enable free movement of healthcare professionals across the EU by ensuring a common core of requirements for countries delivering healthcare programmes; this includes both course content and the number of hours of theory and practice. For nursing, it states that the course should be at least three years in length, or 4,600 hours of study, of which at least half are in practice, hence the requirement from the NMC for courses in the UK to include a minimum of 2,300 hours of practice. As discussed earlier, practice can include learning in skills and simulation, so some of your 2,300 hours may take place in skills laboratories and simulation suites. If you do not know how many hours you will be expected to complete in placements and how many through skills and simulation, check your course handbook or ask your course leader.

The split between placements and skills and simulation will vary between universities, but the majority of your hours will be undertaken in placement settings. You will be required to submit a time sheet (verified by your practice supervisor or assessor) detailing the shifts and hours you have completed in practice for each placement. It will also be a course requirement that you inform both practice and the university if you are absent from practice for any reason as the university has to keep a record of the hours you have completed. Towards the end of your course, the university will check if you are on target to meet the required minimum of 2,300 hours by the end of your programme. If you have had any sickness or absence from practice, you may be required to undertake additional practice hours at the end of the programme to ensure that you have completed the 2,300 hours required to register with the NMC. The university will not be able to sign you off as having completed course requirements until the hours are completed. Your time sheet will also show the range of shifts that you have undertaken over each placement, which is also an important part of meeting your programme requirements.

## Range of practice hours

The NMC expects you to experience the full range of hours that nurses work (e.g. early, late, long days, weekends and night duty). This is important as you need to understand how the work of nursing can vary across the week and through the 24 hours in a day. It is also essential to understanding the patient experience. For example, until you have worked a night shift, it is hard to appreciate fully how a patient may feel if they have had little sleep due to the number of interruptions during the night by staff carrying out care activities, as well as the general noise in the area. Equally, finding out what services and which health and social care staff are available in different healthcare settings across 24 hours a day, seven days a week, is important in informing how you plan patient care, referrals to other services, and discharges. For example, certain services are far more limited at night and at weekends in both hospital and community settings, so planning a discharge for someone on a Friday is not always a good idea if the services they need will not be available until the following Monday. As a student, you will move through different practice areas, which means you will be able to develop an informed perspective on what services are available in both acute and community settings and share these with the people you work with. It is worth checking whether your university stipulates a minimum number of weekends and night shifts to be completed on each placement or over the length of your programme, as this is likely to be a course requirement in order to successfully complete your programme.

## European Working Time Directive

This directive means that you cannot work more than 48 hours a week on average. This is normally averaged over 17 weeks. Some universities may cap your hours as a maximum of 48 hours in any week. It is therefore important to check what the rules are, as if you do exceed these hours, the university may not count them as part of your minimum requirement of 2,300 hours, and you could be in breach of course regulations. It is also important to take this directive into account when planning any paid work you undertake in addition to your placement hours, as excessive hours can impact on your health, and therefore on your performance in university and in practice, as well as potentially on patient safety.

## Range of practice experience

The type and number of placements you will be allocated to will vary depending on the field you are studying, your university's curriculum and how many students each placement can take (placement capacity). For all fields of nursing, the range of experiences usually include placements in acute hospital settings, community settings and settings providing care for people with complex/specialist needs. The university, working with their practice partners, will have developed an agreed pathway of placement experiences for each field of practice and will explain these to you early in your course. You will find that you and your colleagues on the course will not all be allocated experiences in the same order as there will not be enough capacity in each specialism. For example, some students may be allocated to a community placement first and some may undertake a hospital placement first. Some placements may not be suitable for first years, and so will occur later in your programme (e.g. complex care, forensic units). Additionally, students with a disability may require a modified pathway to enable their support needs to be met, and this will be discussed and agreed with them early in their programme. The adjustments that students with a disability may require in practice will be discussed further in Chapter 8.

There are specific requirements regarding the type of placements that students undertaking adult nursing should be allocated to. This is detailed in the *EU Directive 2005/36/EC*, which we discussed earlier. This directive lists the types of placements/clinical experiences a generalist (adult) nurse should gain experience in. The reason they only specify placement experiences for adult nurses is because countries in the EU only train general (or adult) nurses. In many countries in Europe, nurses wishing to specialise in mental health, children's nursing and learning disability nursing usually undertake additional post-registration courses after completing their generalist pre-registration nursing programme.

The required practice experiences for general/adult nurses are:

- general and specialist medicine;
- general and specialist surgery;
- childcare and paediatrics;
- maternity care;
- mental health and psychiatry;
- care of the old and geriatrics; and
- home nursing (in the UK, this would include community nursing, GP practices, health visiting and school nursing).

In some cases, more than one of these experiences can be achieved in one placement allocation. For example, an adult nurse will find older people in most healthcare settings; if you undertake a placement with a health visitor, this covers both home nursing and childcare/paediatrics. However, in the UK, because we have four fields of nursing, there is greater competition for some types of placements. Mental health, paediatrics and maternity have limited capacity and cannot host the significantly larger numbers of adult students, so many universities will offer these experiences through alternative means, such as through skills and simulation and other structured activities in class.

The additional benefits of experiencing a range of different types of placements are that it allows you to work with and learn from a whole variety of people and experience different areas of nursing that will help you decide where you want to work upon registration. Placements are not just about learning from nurses, but also learning from other health and social care professionals. **Person-centred care** requires effective team working across professions, so working with different health and social care professionals will ensure you understand the role each has to play in the provision of care for your patients and service users.

We will look at the allocation process further in the next chapter and explore what you can do if you have a particular difficulty with the type or locality of the placement you have been allocated to.

## Supernumerary status

Supernumerary status can cause confusion and concern for both students and the staff in practice who support them (Shepherd and Uren, 2014); this is because it is often misunderstood. Supernumerary does not mean you don't get involved in patient care; nor does it mean you are there simply to watch and pick and choose what you will do in practice. The NMC has updated its definition of supernumerary status in its latest standards (NMC, 2018d) in order to try to provide more clarity for everyone. Unfortunately, the new definition is quite lengthy, but in essence it is saying that students are not counted as part of the staffing numbers that are required to deliver safe and effective care in a given setting. The NMC reinforces the importance of supernumerary status in its definition, clarifying what supernumerary means for both university-based, self-funding students (they are supernumerary on all placements) and students on an apprenticeship programme (they are supernumerary for specific placement periods/days of the week). We will look at supernumerary status again in Chapter 5 so that you are clear about your rights in practice, the expectations of staff in practice, and what it means for the way you participate in practice settings.

## Practice supervisors and assessors

The NMC sets out its requirements for the learning, support and supervision that will be available to you in the practice environment in its *Standards for Student Supervision and Assessment* (NMC, 2018c). There are two key roles within practice: the practice supervisors, who support you on a day-to-day basis on placement, and the practice asses-sor, who is responsible for confirming that you have met the required proficiencies. We will look at these roles in more detail in Chapter 4.

In addition to the regulatory requirements above, there are a number of guidance documents published by the NMC that have specific relevance to you when on place-ment. They set out best practice and provide details about legislation that you need to be aware of, as well as the support available to you if you are unsure about any aspect contained in the guidance.

# Policies and guidance essential to safe practice

## The Code

*The Code: Professional Standards of Practice and Behaviour for Nurses, Midwives and Nursing Associates* (NMC, 2018a) is an essential guide for you as a student when in practice. It sets out the professional standards that registered nurses, midwives and nursing associates are required to uphold, and applies to all registrants in whatever setting they work in, as well as how they conduct certain aspects of their personal life. As a student, it provides you with an insight into the expectations of the professional role of the nurse, and therefore the expectations that patients, service users and carers, as well as the people you work with, will also have of you. The standards set out the key principles and expectations of the values and behav-iours registrants must demonstrate when providing care and provide you with an understanding of what good practice looks like. While all the standards are impor-tant, some of them are particularly important for you to appreciate as a student going out on placement.

## Consent

While most patients and service users are very happy for students to be involved in their care, there will be occasions when they may refuse your involvement, and they have the right to do so. You should not take this personally. Sometimes it will be because they do not understand your role or are not aware that you are under supervision and will not be undertaking any care activity unless the person super-vising you is confident that you are competent to do so. It is therefore important that when you are in practice, the people you care for are always informed that you are a student and are given the opportunity to withdraw their consent to you being involved in their care (NMC, 2018b). It is also essential that even when you have informed someone before that you are a student, you still seek consent before you undertake any care activities with them in the future, as required by *The Code* (NMC, 2018a).

# Confidentiality and data protection

You will be privy to very personal information about the people in your care, and it is essential that you do not share this information inappropriately. Patients and service users will provide you with a lot of personal information about themselves when you are undertaking admissions assessments and while you are delivering care to them. You will also have access to their nursing and medical notes, which will contain very personal and detailed information; all of this information is confidential. Section 5 of *The Code* (NMC, 2018a) provides guidance on maintaining confidentiality in practice, but if you are ever unsure about information that you have been given by a patient or service user and who you can share it with, it is essential that you seek advice from a qualified member of staff on your placement.

While in practice, it is likely that you will be provided with a swipe or smart card to access **electronic patient records** for the people in your care. It is important that you keep this secure and do not allow anyone else to use it. Read the case study below, which explores this aspect of practice in more detail, before attempting Activity 1.3.

---

## Case study: Gemma

Gemma has been allocated to a ward in her local hospital. She has a smart card to access patient records on her placement and decides to look up details regarding one of her relatives on the hospital system. The hospital picks up the unusual access activity and is able to track who has made the data access and reports this to the university. Gemma is referred for a **fitness to practise** hearing.

---

## Activity 1.3   Critical thinking

Why do you think Gemma was referred to a fitness to practise hearing?

*An outline answer to this activity is given at the end of the chapter.*

---

For Gemma, there were serious consequences to her actions. You will receive training on **information governance and data security** as part of your course to ensure that you are fully aware of your responsibilities and do not find yourself in a situation like Gemma's.

# Social media

Social media is widely used to connect people and share news, personal views, ideas, photos and videos via the Internet. It encompasses a wide range of Internet-based platforms; examples of some of these are shown in Figure 1.3.

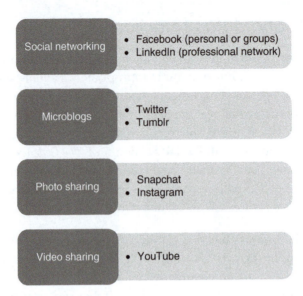

*Figure 1.3* Examples of social media

It is highly likely that you are familiar with and use at least one of these Internet platforms, and that is absolutely fine (even the NMC uses social media), but as a student nurse you must ensure that you use these platforms responsibly and ensure that people's privacy is respected at all times (NMC, 2018a).

One of the benefits and problems with social media is the speed with which information can be shared and disseminated. You may post something on Facebook, for example, which you believe only your friends and family can see. However, the information or photos that you post can be copied and shared by them, and it is then quickly available to people outside your immediate circle.

The same applies to texts or the use of phone applications such as WhatsApp or Facebook Messenger, where messages can very quickly be disseminated between people.

The NMC's *Guidance on Using Social Media Responsibly* (NMC, 2017a) applies *The Code* to the use of social media. The guidance provides examples of where use of social media can be deemed as inappropriate, unprofessional or even unlawful, and could lead to a registrant being removed from the NMC register or a student being withdrawn from their course. Table 1.2 lists some of the actions that could put your place on the course at risk.

| Sharing confidential information inappropriately |
| --- |
| Posting pictures of patients and people receiving care without their consent |
| Posting inappropriate comments about patients |
| Bullying, intimidating or exploiting people |
| Building or pursuing relationships with patients or service users |

| Stealing personal information or using someone else's identity |
| Encouraging violence or self-harm |
| Inciting hatred or discrimination |

*Table 1.2*   Unprofessional or unlawful use of social media

*Source*: NMC (2017a, p3)

Posting a derogatory comment about a patient or members of staff you are working with, even if you don't name them, would be seen as unprofessional, as would posting photos of yourself in your uniform in inappropriate poses, or 'liking' a photo on Facebook where the photo may be seen as discriminatory. Activity 1.4 provides you with some case studies from the NMC website where registrants have been referred to them due to concerns regarding their fitness to practise.

## Activity 1.4   Reflection

**NMC conduct and competence committee hearings**

Go to the NMC website (**www.nmc.org.uk**) and use the search function on their website to search for cases regarding inappropriate use of social media by using the case numbers below:

- 35146;
- 057619; and
- 48544.

Are you surprised at the penalty applied in each of these cases?

Consider the comments that these registrants made on social media. Looking at your own use of social media, have you ever posted anything on social media, or commented on photos, videos or news items posted on social media, that on reflection you believe now may be inappropriate?

*As this activity is based on your own observation, there is no outline answer at the end of the chapter.*

It is important to put all of this into context. The number of registrants referred to the NMC due to inappropriate use of social media is low, with six social media cases out of a total of 706 fitness to practise cases between 2016 and 2017 (NMC, 2017b), and social media offers lots of positives for you as a student; you just need to consider very carefully what you post or comment on. If a friend or colleague makes a comment that appears on your social media page that is inappropriate, you can ask them to remove it, or you can usually delete it from your own page.

There are, however, a number of benefits in using social media as a student nurse that will help you on your course; some examples of accounts you may find of interest are listed in Table 1.3 to get you started.

| Type | Name | Link/Twitter handle |
|---|---|---|
| Twitter | RCN Students – RCN student committee | @RCNStudents |
| Twitter | WeNurses – regular scheduled chats by healthcare professionals | @WeNurses @WeStudentNurse @WeCYPNurses @WeLDnurses @WeMHnurses www.wecommunities.org |
| Twitter | The NMC | @nmcnews |
| Blog | nhsManagers.net – a daily e-letter from Roy Lilley related to the NHS | https://ihm.org.uk/roy-lilley-nhsmanagers/ |
| Blog and Twitter | The Student Nurse Project | https://studentnurseproject.co.uk @StNurseProject |
| Facebook | Royal College of Nursing Students | www.facebook.com/RCNStudents/ |

*Table 1.3* Social media sites

Social media offers an opportunity to link with colleagues in your cohort, but also with peers from across the country/world, and share best practice, pose questions and keep up to date on new innovations, conferences and publications, and so on. Start by joining a well-recognised group that will have a moderator overseeing the suitability of the posts/photos and become familiar with the types of posts members send, as well as the range of topics discussed, before stepping in yourself with your own views and ideas. Remember that when you do start to post anything as a student nurse, it is also as a student of your university, so at all times consider the appropriateness of what you post, and if in doubt seek guidance from your personal tutor or a member of staff from the university.

## Scenario: Facebook

Sasha, a friend of yours, takes a photo of a new lecturer using her phone during class and posts it on your cohort's Facebook page. She comments on his good looks, and some of the other students on your course join in with more comments.

Consider Sasha's behaviour in the above scenario to help you complete Activity 1.5.

## Activity 1.5   Reflection

Review the NMC's *Guidance on Using Social Media Responsibly* (NMC, 2017a) and think about the below questions in relation to Sasha's behaviour:

1.   What are the issues raised in this scenario?
2.   How might you respond?

*An outline answer to this activity is given at the end of the chapter.*

While taking a photo of a member of staff and making a comment about them may not be seen as very serious, it does question Sasha's understanding of professional behaviour. Both the university and the practice partners who provide your placements will have very high expectations of your behaviour, so let's explore these expectations further.

# The expectations of the university and placement providers

In exploring the regulations, standards and guides developed by the NMC above, one concept is a constant theme: professionalism. It is also seen as an essential behaviour by both your university and their practice partners. The term 'professional' is widely used, but a clear definition of what professionalism means specifically for nurses and midwives had not been clearly articulated until 2017, when the NMC published the framework *Enabling Professionalism in Nursing and Midwifery Practice* (NMC, 2017c). This framework is underpinned by *The Code* to clarify what professionalism means and how it can be enacted and supported in practice.

The NMC defines professionalism in nursing and midwifery as being:

> *characterised by the autonomous evidence-based decision making by members of an occupation who share the same values and education. Professionalism in nursing and midwifery is realised through purposeful relationships and underpinned by environments that facilitate professional practice. Professional nurses and midwives demonstrate and embrace accountability for their actions.*

(NMC, 2017c, p3)

So, from an NMC perspective, professionalism is not just about you and how you behave, but also about how the environments in which you work help you to develop and maintain professionalism. From a student perspective, this means both at university and out on placement. The framework describes:

- the purpose of professionalism;
- the attributes that demonstrate professionalism;
- organisational and environmental factors to support and enable professional practice and behaviours; and
- individual responsibilities to support and enable professional practice and behaviours.

(NMC, 2017c, p2)

While the main focus is on the registered nurse or midwife it is an important guide for you as a student in understanding what is and will be expected of you as you progress through the course. However, the staff in practice and at university will also have some very specific expectations of you that they will see as important in demonstrating professionalism. For example:

- demonstrating appropriate personal presentation and adherence to the dress code;
- demonstrating punctuality and informing practice/university if unable to attend;
- engaging positively in all learning opportunities;
- recognising and working within your own limitations of knowledge and skills, and seeking support and advice when appropriate;
- demonstrating person-centred, compassionate care;
- maintaining professional boundaries;
- reporting any concerns to a member of staff when appropriate;
- adhering to *The Code* and local policies and procedures;
- reflecting on learning; and
- providing feedback on learning experiences.

We will pick up on many of these points in the next couple of chapters when we look at how to prepare for a practice placement and how to maximise your learning in practice.

## Chapter summary

This chapter has explored what is meant by practice, emphasising the importance of both practice placements and skills and simulation in enabling you to develop the skills and knowledge to meet the NMC standards and proficiencies and register as a nurse. The structure and requirements for practice are guided by both EU directives and NMC standards, with many elements non-negotiable in order to achieve

NMC requirements. The NMC has published a number of standards and guidelines that nurses and nursing students are expected to follow to ensure safe, person-centred care based on best practice. In some situations, such as informed consent, confidentiality and data protection, the student is under a legal obligation to ensure that their actions are lawful. Practice is essential in developing your professional identity as a nurse and entails a socialisation process that will mould your values, beliefs and behaviours, as well as enabling you to demonstrate the professionalism expected by both the university and practice partners.

## Activities: brief outline answers

### Activity 1.2   Critical thinking (p7)

The university requires students to adhere to the dress code when in skills and simulation labs as your time there is about developing your understanding of what it means to be professional in your practice, which is not just about what you know and what you do, but also about how you present yourself. All of these elements are important in developing trust with the patients and carers you will be coming into contact with in practice. It is also linked with university and practice partner expectations of you. In Rosa's case, this is also about health and safety. In the skills labs, you will be practising skills on your colleagues and role players, and false nails can scratch people, prevent you from washing your hands thoroughly, and harbour bacteria, and so pose an infection risk (Infection Control Team, 2016). Therefore, the standards expected of you in skills and simulation will be the same as when you are in practice, and your time in the skills labs will help you to understand why these standards are expected of you.

### Activity 1.3   Critical thinking (p13)

Patients provide very personal information, and in doing so trust that their information will be kept secure and only shared with those directly involved in their care. Gemma has breached patient trust and confidentiality in accessing these records, and so is in breach of *The Code* as well as the Data Protection Act 2018. In addition, Gemma could be taken to court. The Information Commissioner's Office (ICO) records examples of cases of illegal access here: **https://tinyurl. com/illegal-access**

### Activity 1.5   Reflection (p17)

The possible issues relate to the invasion of the lecturer's privacy if his consent was not sought, as well as the distress to the lecturer if he found out that he had been the subject of a discussion about his appearance. Taking the lecturer's photo without his permission and posting it on Facebook is likely to be viewed as professional misconduct by the university.

Possible responses to this situation for you would be asking the student who posted the photo to remove it or seeking advice from your personal tutor.

## Further reading

**Delves-Yates, C., Everett, F. and Wright, W.** (2018) *Essential Clinical Skills for Nurses: Step by Step.* London: SAGE.

Covers core skills that can help you prepare for skills and simulation or practice.

**Royal College of Nursing (RCN)** (2017) *Helping Students Get the Best from Their Practice Placements: A Royal College of Nursing Toolkit.* London: RCN.

Explains the importance of practice placements and provides useful tips.

## Useful websites

Nursing and Midwifery Standards

**www.nmc.org.uk/standards/**

This web page contains the education standards related to your programme, as well as *The Code* and additional guidance documents discussed in this chapter.

Royal College of Nursing Advice Guides for Students

**www.rcn.org.uk/get-help/rcn-advice/student-nurses**

A series of short guides for student nurses on a range of topics, including placements, accountability and raising concerns.

We Communities

**www.wecommunities.org**

Hosts a number of nursing Twitter chat groups and a range of resources on using social media.

# Chapter 2

# Preparing for your placement

Karen Elcock

## NMC Standards of Proficiency for Registered Nurses

This chapter will address the following platforms and proficiencies:

**Platform 1: Being an accountable professional**

Registered nurses act in the best interests of people, putting them first and providing nursing care that is person-centred, safe and compassionate. They act professionally at all times and use their knowledge and experience to make evidence-based decisions about care. They communicate effectively, are role models for others, and are accountable for their actions. Registered nurses continually reflect on their practice and keep abreast of new and emerging developments in nursing, health and care.

At the point of registration, the registered nurse will be able to:

1.1 understand and act in accordance with *The Code: Professional Standards of Practice and Behaviour for Nurses, Midwives and Nursing Associates,* and fulfil all registration requirements.

1.2 understand and apply relevant legal, regulatory and governance requirements, policies, and ethical frameworks, including any mandatory reporting duties, to all areas of practice, differentiating where appropriate between the devolved legislatures of the United Kingdom.

1.5 understand the demands of professional practice and demonstrate how to recognise signs of vulnerability in themselves or their colleagues and the action required to minimise risks to health.

**Platform 4: Providing and evaluating care**

Registered nurses take the lead in providing evidence-based, compassionate and safe nursing interventions. They ensure that care they provide and delegate is person-centred

*(Continued)*

(Continued)

and of a consistently high standard. They support people of all ages in a range of care settings. They work in partnership with people, families and carers to evaluate whether care is effective and the goals of care have been met in line with their wishes, preferences and desired outcomes.

At the point of registration, the registered nurse will be able to:

4.12 demonstrate the ability to manage commonly encountered devices and confidently carry out related nursing procedures to meet people's needs for evidence-based, person-centred care.

4.13 demonstrate the knowledge, skills and confidence to provide first aid procedures and basic life support.

**Platform 6: Improving safety and quality of care**

Registered nurses make a key contribution to the continuous monitoring and quality improvement of care and treatment in order to enhance health outcomes and people's experience of nursing and related care. They assess risks to safety or experience and take appropriate action to manage those, putting the best interests, needs and preferences of people first.

At the point of registration, the registered nurse will be able to:

6.1 understand and apply the principles of health and safety legislation and regulations and maintain safe work and care environments.

6.3 comply with local and national frameworks, legislation and regulations for assessing, managing and reporting risks, ensuring the appropriate action is taken.

## Chapter aims

After reading this chapter, you will be able to:

* appreciate how placements are allocated;
* outline the different types of placements you will be allocated to and the implications for your planning and preparation;
* investigate, using a range of resources, to develop an understanding of the organisations you are allocated to;

- consider the different factors that you need to consider in travelling to your placement and balancing personal/family needs with course/placement requirements;
- describe the process for making first contact with your placement; and
- understand what the prerequisites are before you can attend placement, and why.

# Introduction

Preparation for your placement is essential in order to ensure you are prepared to deliver safe and effective care and to enable you to maximise your learning experiences in practice. Preparation for practice is equally important for every placement you undertake, not just your first one. This chapter will look at a range of activities you can undertake in preparing for your placements, starting with a consideration of the basics, such as how to contact your placement and how you will get there. You will also be asked to consider how you will manage any personal and family needs in order to meet the demands of the placement. The importance of finding out what learning opportunities the placement will offer you will be explored so that you can reflect on what you already know and what you will need to learn about. This will guide you in identifying what learning activities you can undertake to become familiar with the needs of the client group and placement type, which will enable you to feel better prepared and provide a smooth transition into your placement.

# The placement allocation process

Many universities will allocate students to a zone, or geographical area, often based around one or more NHS trusts. In some parts of the UK, the zone can cover a wide geographical area to ensure you get the range of experiences you will need to meet NMC requirements. If you have already completed Activity 1.1 in Chapter 1, then you will already know who the organisations are that provide placements for your university; if not, go back and complete the activity now. You will be informed about the number and different types of placements (often called placement pathways) you will be allocated to over the course of your programme early in your course. Commonly, there are two or three placements per year, and the range will incorporate at least one in-patient (hospital-based) placement, a community placement and a placement that involves caring for people with complex, specialist or high-dependency needs. In addition, you will also gain experience in what may be called interface placements, where patients may require a short episode of care, or within an organisation that sits between a hospital and the community. As we discussed in Chapter 1, adult nursing students require very specific types of placement to meet EU and NMC requirements; however, for the other fields, there is no pre-scribed placement pathway. Different placement pathways for each field of nursing are shown in Table 2.1, with examples of the different types of placements within each pathway. These are not exhaustive, and you may gain experience in additional areas not listed below.

| Field | Placement types with examples |
|---|---|
| **Adult** | **Surgical** (e.g. surgical wards, ear, nose and throat, orthopaedic, cardiothoracic, urology, gynaecology, ophthalmology, general surgery, day surgery units, theatres and recovery) |
| | **Medical wards** (e.g. cardiology, respiratory, rheumatology, neurology, infectious diseases, oncology, haematology, HIV/AIDS, rheumatology, general medicine, elderly care wards) |
| | **Complex care** (e.g. accident and emergency, high-dependency unit, intensive care unit/intensive therapy unit, acute medical unit, acute admissions unit, coronary care unit, surgical assessment unit) |
| | **Community** (e.g. district nurse, primary care, GP practice, health visitor, community hospitals, community matron, sexual health clinics) |
| | **Interface** (e.g. hospice, rehabilitation units, dialysis units, endoscopy, outpatient department, walk-in centre, minor injuries unit, nursing homes) |
| **Child** | **Acute inpatient hospital** (e.g. general and specialist surgical wards, surgical day care, medical wards often dealing with chronic/long-term conditions) |
| | **Community** (e.g. health visitor, community children's team, school nurse, community matron) |
| | **Interface** (e.g. children's hospice, day-care surgery, assessment unit, outpatient department, specialist residential and community-based rehabilitation services, respite/short-break services, special schools) |
| | **Complex care** (e.g. high-dependency unit, paediatric intensive care unit, neonatal intensive care unit, special care baby unit, accident and emergency, child and adolescent mental health teams) |
| **Learning disability** | **Community learning disability team** |
| | **Community services for children** (e.g. child and adolescent mental health teams, children and young people services) |
| | **Children or adults with acute/complex healthcare needs** |
| | **Education** (e.g. special schools or FE colleges) |
| | **Acute mental health or specialist learning disability assessment/treatment units** |
| **Mental health** | **Acute inpatient** (including recovery unit, complex care and dementia wards) |
| | **Community** (e.g. home treatment teams, community mental health teams, community complex care, dementia) |
| | **Specialist community** (e.g. drug and alcohol recovery team, forensic community mental health teams, early intervention services, older people) |
| | **Specialist services** (e.g. child and adolescent mental health teams, forensic/low-secure units, eating disorder services, prisons, recovery, older people, acute psychiatric liaison, psychiatric intensive care units, deaf adult services) |

*Table 2.1* Placement pathways

As you can see, there are a huge variety of placements. While it is not possible to experience all of these, you will probably experience at least one from each of the placement pathway types shown, depending on the availability of services in your area and the pathways designed by your university. In addition, at some universities, you may be allocated what are commonly called insight placements, in one or more of the other fields of nursing. Another type of placement allocation is the 'hub-and-spoke' placement. On these placements, you will have a main home or hub placement but will spend from one to four weeks in other areas (the spokes), which are related to the needs of your patient/service users and provide an insight into their journey through the healthcare system (Thomas and Westwood, 2016). Some placements provide a modified form of hub-and-spoke placement by offering outreach placements that are much shorter in length (e.g. half a day or possibly a couple of days). These outreach placements will give you an insight into different departments a patient/service user may visit during their hospital stay or enable you to spend time with different health and social care professionals in hospitals, or in the community who provide care to your client group. Regardless of the format of your placement, the university will ensure you get a breadth of experience that will enable you to meet both NMC and course requirements. Read the following scenario about Josh's reaction to his placement allocation and then answer the questions in Activity 2.1.

---

## Scenario: Josh's disappointment

Imagine that you have a friend called Josh on the course who has chosen nursing as a career because he wanted to work with people with drug and alcohol addiction, having seen how these addictions have impacted on friends and families. Josh had undertaken a lot of research into this area prior to applying for nursing and had decided what type of placements he wanted to do on his course to enable him to get a job in this field when he qualified. He was very upset when he found out that he could not have all the placements on his list and said he was thinking of dropping out of the programme if the university could not give him what he wanted.

---

## Activity 2.1   Critical thinking

What advice might you offer Josh?

*An outline answer to this activity is given at the end of the chapter.*

Josh could also consider taking his elective in a placement that provides services for people with drug and alcohol issues. Most universities now offer students an opportunity to undertake an elective at some point in their programme in addition to the main placement areas in a field pathway, as we discussed earlier. An elective can provide you with an opportunity to gain experience of nursing abroad, somewhere else in the UK or in an area of practice that won't be available to you via your university, as has occurred for Josh. We will look at electives in more detail in Chapter 7.

Unsurprisingly, the allocation of students is complex, and while the university will endeavour to allocate you to placements within a reasonable distance from home, sometimes you will be required to travel further in order to access placements that ensure you meet the range required to meet programme and NMC requirements. It is therefore important for you to consider how you will get to each of your placements well in advance of the first day.

# Travelling to your placement

You may not yet have considered how you will get to your placement or maybe thought you would just catch a bus. However, thinking about how you will travel to your placement is not just considering the mode of transport, but also considering how you will get to your placement for different shifts, as well as at weekends and bank holidays. Activity 2.2 asks you to research journey times to your placement. If you don't yet know where you will be placed, you could use the postcodes of one of the key hospital trusts or organisations that your university offers placements at as a starting point.

## Activity 2.2    Research

Look up the postcode of an organisation that will be providing you with placements as part of your university course. Use Google Maps to search for the journey options using your home/accommodation postcode and the placement postcode. You can refine your search to look at journey times using public transport, a car, bicycle or walking, as well as specifying the dates and times you want to arrive or leave by. Now check the journey times for:

1.  Arriving at your placement at least 15 minutes before the start of an early shift (or long day) and then the start of a late shift on a weekday. Repeat for a Saturday and a Sunday.
2.  Leaving your placement at the end of a late shift (or long day) on a weekday, a Saturday and a Sunday.

*As this activity is based on your own observation, there is no outline answer at the end of the chapter.*

Depending on your mode of transport you may or may not have been surprised by the results of this activity. If using public transport, you may have found that some journeys are difficult or even impossible (e.g. on Sundays or bank holidays) and that some journey times vary depending on when your shift starts or ends. It is therefore important that you let your university know as soon as possible if you think there will be problems for you to get to your allocated placement so that they can explore the options available to you. Depending on where you live, which university you are at and the time of day you are travelling, travel times can sometimes take up to two hours each way. It is therefore important to fully research the different travel options against the different start and end times for each of the different types of shifts you will be asked to undertake so that you are sure that you can undertake the full range a placement rosters you for. Wherever possible, the university will take into account where you are living when allocating your placements, so it is essential that you keep your university informed if you change address. If you do find that travel to and from a placement is particularly difficult, you may be able to claim for overnight accommodation, but do seek advice on the process for this at your university before booking it.

In addition to looking at travel times, it is also essential to consider your personal safety as you will be travelling early in the morning and late at night, which in winter means travelling in the dark. A personal alarm is a good buy. The British Council website has some valuable tips on travelling safety using public transport: **http:// esol.britishcouncil.org/content/learners/uk-life/be-safe-uk/staying-safe-public-transport**

# Getting to know your placement

One way to impress your placement is to show that you have undertaken some preparatory work to find out about the organisation and the placement itself. There are a number of sources you can access via the Internet to do this:

- The first stop is your own university website as many now have detailed information on their placements, including contacts, shifts, travel guides, learning opportunities, expectations of students and induction packs for the placement.
- The organisation's own website is a great starting point. Most organisations will have, at a minimum, contact details, instructions on how to get there, their visions

and values, key strategies, and news items, all of which can give you an insight and feel about the organisation. Larger organisations such as NHS trusts will often have details about individual wards or services and key staff that will give you further insight into your placement.

- The Care Quality Commission (CQC) is an independent regulator of health and adult social care in England. They have a number of roles, but their key role is to monitor, inspect and rate services and publish reports on their website, which you (and the public) can download and read. These reports will provide you with information on what the organisation you are being placed at does well and areas they may have for improvement and may also include information about your specific placement.

- If your placement is at an NHS trust, you can search for details about the trust on the NHS website (**www.nhs.uk**). This site provides an overview of the organisation, details about the wards and services, contact details, and maps. You can also read ratings and reviews left by people who have used the service, as well as the organisation's CQC report, and the scores they have received for their Friends and Family Test (FFT), including specific departments within the organisation.

- The FFT provides the people who use NHS services an opportunity to give feedback on their experience (see **www.england.nhs.uk/fft/**). The questionnaire asks whether they would recommend the services they have used to friends or family if they needed similar care or treatment, and also offers an opportunity for them to give additional and more detailed feedback if they wish to. Similar surveys are carried out in Scotland (Scottish Care Experience Survey Programme), Wales (patient satisfaction surveys) and Northern Ireland (patient experience surveys). In addition, the NHS also undertakes a staff survey once a year to allow staff to give their feedback on the organisation they work at, which you can also access on the Internet at: **www.nhsstaffsurveys.com/**

Accessing the above resources will not only offer you an insight into your placement, but also provide you with information that will be useful in helping you make contact with and plan your journey to the placement. Most non-NHS organisations also have websites that will provide you with a range of information that will also be useful in planning for your placement, including CQC reports, or Ofsted reports if they are an educational institution.

A note of caution, though. Many CQC reports will identify areas for improvement, which is part of their role. If you have any concerns, do talk them through with your personal tutor. Universities work closely with their practice partners and will review CQC visits to ensure that there are no issues for the quality of student learning.

# Learning about the placement speciality

In addition to gaining an understanding about the organisation in which you have been placed, it is important to read around the speciality in the specific placement you have been allocated to. Activity 2.3 asks you to consider how you would do this.

---

### Activity 2.3   Critical thinking

Imagine you have just received details about your placement. What preparation would you undertake to ensure you understand more about the speciality it offers?

*An outline answer to this activity is given at the end of the chapter.*

---

Reading and research are fundamental to success when studying for a degree and should not be seen as something you just do to prepare for an assignment. To get the most out of each placement, it is essential that you research the speciality and read around the relevant topics related to your placement. This will help you to feel more confident when you start as you will be more familiar with the terminology that staff use (a crib list of key terms and abbreviations is always useful to take with you). It will also help you to maximise your learning from the placement as you will have greater insight into what learning opportunities are available to you and also help you to improve the care you give while there, as you will be basing it on the evidence you have read. An added bonus is that reading around the learning opportunities and specialisms your placement offers can have a positive impact on your assignments, as you link theory and practice through your reading, research and practice experiences. We will look at this again in more detail in Chapter 5.

# Making first contact with your placement

---

### Research summary: Getting there

A study undertaken in Scotland explored nursing students' experience of placements (MacDonald et al., 2016). One of the findings was called 'getting there' and explored the students' experience of preparing for and contacting their placement. Students found the process intimidating, with practical worries about how to get there, wondering how much food to take for a 12-hour shift, and the anxieties of phoning a placement and not getting through, or finding that they are not expected or their off-duty is not yet organised. As one student said, 'This is the first impression of the practice area and that experience can either instil panic or provide reassurance' (p46).

---

It is not only how prepared the ward is for you, but also the impression you make in how you make contact, that will have an impact on how you settle into your placement. It is therefore important to try to ring up at least a couple of weeks before you are due to start, unless your university advises differently; this will allow time for both you and the placement to be properly prepared for your start. Read the case study about Aoife's experience of contacting her placement and then complete Activity 2.4.

---

## Case study: Aoife

Aoife has received the details of her placement and rings the ward. The ward clerk answers and says that the staff are busy, and she should ring back later. Aoife is in class, so rings back the next day and manages to talk to a nurse, who says she is not sure what has been organised and suggests that it is best if she just turns up on the first day and that everything will be organised once she gets there. Aoife doesn't want to make a fuss so says, 'OK' and puts the phone down. She feels deflated and is now very anxious about her placement.

---

## Activity 2.4   Critical thinking

Imagine you are Aoife. How might you have managed this differently? What problems might a response such as this cause you?

*An outline answer to this activity is given at the end of the chapter.*

---

This was not a good start for Aoife, but unfortunately this does happen sometimes, and when the response is not what you expect it can throw you off course, so you forget to ask what you needed to know. Before contacting your placement, make a list of what you need to ask as this will keep you focused. Questions you should consider are:

- The name of the person you are talking to. This makes it more personal, but also if there are any queries later you can refer back to the person you talked to.
- What shift patterns are you expected to work? Long days or short days? Do they include weekends or night duty, and what time do they start and finish?
- What is your **rota** for the first week, and what time do they want you to arrive on the first day?
- Are you required to wear uniform, and if so is there anywhere to get changed at the placement?
- What are the names of your practice assessor and practice supervisor, and who will be your key contact for the first day?

- Who is the nurse/person in charge?
- Have they got an **induction booklet** for students that they could send you before you start so you can do some preparation?

If the information was not provided by your university, you also need to know who the contact person from your university is for your placement.

## Negotiating shifts

You will be expected to undertake the same shift pattern as staff within your placement area. Your rota will usually be planned so that you are working with staff who can supervise your learning and provide you with the opportunity to maximise the learning opportunities on placement. However, there is scope for some negotiation in your shifts, which you will need to discuss with your practice supervisor or assessor in placement. The university may have rules regarding how many weekends and night shifts you should undertake during your course, so you will need to ensure you meet these requirements in order to meet the NMC's programme standards that you experience the range of hours that nurses work.

## Reasonable adjustments

If you have any reasonable adjustments that need to be put in place while on placement, you will need to disclose these to at least one person on your placement so they can ensure that they can be met. Depending on the adjustments required, it can be helpful to visit your placement in advance of your start date to discuss what your needs are. Chapter 8 will look at reasonable adjustments in more detail.

# Common fears and anxieties

Going out on placement causes both anxieties and excitement. A small-scale research study involving first-year child field students in the UK explored their anxieties prior to going out on their first placement (Brady et al., 2017), which are shown in Table 2.2. Reflect on these anxieties and then complete Activity 2.5.

| Excitement | Visiting the placement, learning about the children they will be caring for |
|---|---|
| Anxiety | How parents and children will perceive them, not being a burden, not learning enough, completing the practice assessment document |
| Concerns | Fitting in, getting on with their mentor, appearing professional, not wanting to make mistakes |
| Ownership | Talking about 'my mentor', my placement', 'my ward' |
| Use of jargon | Understanding new and unfamiliar terms used in practice |

*Table 2.2*  Students' anxieties and concerns prior to their first placement

*Source*: Brady et al. (2017)

## Activity 2.5   Reflection

How do the anxieties and concerns listed in Table 2.2 compare with your own about going out to practice?

*As this activity is based on your own reflection, there is no outline answer at the end of the chapter.*

Many of these anxieties and concerns are not specific to the first placement; they will be experienced prior to every placement as each is new, and so to a degree unknown. The need to 'fit in' and have a sense of 'belongingness' on placement are common to many students. Dunbar and Carter (2017) describe how this need to feel you belong (of feeling 'at home' on a placement) is so important to students that fitting in is often prioritised over other requirements for a placement, such as your personal learning needs. However, if you feel at home and part of the team, then you will feel more able to ask questions, share concerns and seek support, all of which are important if you are to get the most out of your placement.

Table 2.3 lists the resources (ranked in order with the most important at the top) that helped first-year students to prepare for their first placement. Look at the ranking and consider whether you agree, and then complete Activity 2.6.

| Resources that helped students to prepare for their first placement | |
| --- | --- |
| Talk by a student from Year 2 | Most useful |
| Pre-visit to placement and phone call | |
| Peer support and helpful tips | |
| Placement website | |
| Zone induction (induction to the organisation) | |
| Advice from lecturers about being open-minded | |
| Finding out what specialist services are involved | |
| Speaking to my personal tutor or another lecturer about my anxieties | |
| Having a student from the same cohort in the same placement (beforehand) | Least useful |

*Table 2.3*   Preparing for the first placement

*Source*: Brady et al. (2017)

Visiting your placement before starting can be very helpful as it gives you a dry run on how to get there, how long it takes and how to find the actual placement itself; you will also have an idea of where to go once you get to the ward/unit/practice you are placed at. Some placements provide an induction pack for students, and this can be very helpful in explaining more about the potential learning opportunities available to you, as well as providing details of some pre-reading you can undertake that will help you understand more about the client group you will be caring for. Discussing your fears and anxieties with your peers is also helpful as they will have similar feelings about their placement and knowing this can help. While speaking to their personal tutor was low down in the list of resources students accessed in Table 2.3, it can be helpful to talk your anxieties through with them, as they may be able to offer additional advice or offer coping strategies that you can use to help you through those first few days.

# Prerequisites before attending placement

Prior to attending your first placement, you will need to have received occupational health clearance, including all required vaccinations, and have had your criminal record check completed and returned through your country-specific **Disclosure and Barring Service (DBS)**. These checks are a requirement by the NMC (2018d) to ensure that you are of sufficient good health and good character to ensure protection of the public. Having a criminal conviction or declaring a health condition or disability will not necessarily prevent you from becoming a nurse, but failing to declare them to the university could, as failure to declare either a health condition/disability or previous convictions will lead to doubts about your honesty and integrity. The public needs to have trust in you as a nurse, and so if you declare or are found to have a prior conviction the university will need to determine your suitability to remain on the programme.

If you have a health condition or disability, the university will refer you to the occupational health team, who will decide whether you are fit to study and attend practice, and if so whether any adjustments are required while at the university or when on placement. A referral to the disability team will mean that any reasonable adjustments you require can be identified and put in place. These adjustments are important to ensure that you can practise safely and effectively, as well as ensuring that you are not substantially disadvantaged in your studies or while learning in practice.

In addition to good health and a good character check, you will be expected to have completed a number of core mandatory skills.

## Statutory and mandatory training

You will be required to complete core health and safety training prior to attending practice, which take place either in the skills and simulation laboratories or in class or through online activities/modules. These may be called statutory or mandatory training. Statutory training is required by law (e.g. the Health and Safety at Work Act 1974) and is compulsory, whereas mandatory training covers areas that the placement providers have determined as compulsory to ensure safe and effective practice, which are specific to organisational needs and policies (RCN, 2018a). These sessions are essential to prepare you for practice but will also ensure that you can keep yourself, your colleagues in practice and the people in your care safe. Activity 2.7 asks you to find out what your university offers.

### Activity 2.7   Research

Look at your course/practice handbook or on your virtual learning environment to identify what statutory and mandatory training is required at your university prior to commencing placement.

*An outline of possible answers can be found at the end of the chapter.*

The list provided at the end of the chapter is not exhaustive, and there may be additional sessions that will occur throughout your course or be built upon each year so that all elements are completed by the end of your programme. In addition, some have to be repeated every year, such as moving and handling, resuscitation, and information governance and data security. Your university will ensure that this is set up for you each year.

## The Practice Assessment Document

Universities will use different terms for the document that contains the skills and knowledge that you will be assessed on for each placement, but the **Practice Assessment Document (PAD)** is a common one. An **Ongoing Achievement Record**

**(OAR)** may be part of your PAD or an additional document. Both are essential to each placement as they will have to be completed by your practice supervisors and assessors to evidence the skills and knowledge you have achieved on your placement.

Prior to each placement, it is essential that you have read through your PAD and familiarised yourself with the contents, as well as what sections have to be completed by whom and by when. If your university provides you with a hard-copy document, then sticking Post-it notes in each section that needs completing is a good reminder to ensure you get all the parts completed. If you have an electronic document, you may be able to download it and annotate it on your computer/tablet/phone. Think about the type of placement you are going to and identify which skills/proficiencies in your assessment document you think you could achieve there. Make a note of which ones you want to focus on so that you can discuss them with your practice supervisor/assessor in your first week. Showing you have thought about what you need to do while on your placement will show that you are interested and engaged with the learning process, which means staff will invest more of their time in supporting your learning. Chapter 6 looks at the assessment process in more detail.

# Planning your work-life balance

In addition to planning for your placement, it is essential that you also consider how you will manage your work-life balance. As a student nurse, you face far more challenges than a student who is undertaking a standard degree course. Your university year is longer, and in addition to studying for your degree you have to complete a minimum of 2,300 hours of practice. Often you will find yourself studying and writing assignments while on placement. Balancing the day-to-day demands that attending placement make on you in terms of time (travelling and long shifts), the psychological demands in caring for people who are seriously ill or in distress, and the physical demands of long hours and being on your feet for long periods is challenging. If you are also undertaking paid work and/or have caring duties for family or children, then these are additional demands not only on your time, but also on your physical and mental well-being. It is therefore essential to plan how you will meet these different demands, as well as planning in time for yourself. Chapter 3 explores the concept of resilience and will help you to recognise and manage both immediate and long-term pressures on your course, as well as looking at strategies to help you manage them.

# How preparation for practice differs for apprentices

If you are on an apprenticeship programme, preparing for practice may be a little different for you. The majority of your learning will usually occur in the organisation where you are an apprentice, which means you will have undertaken an induction to the organisation and be familiar with how the organisation works. However, the NMC requirement that you have a range of different experiences in clinical practice will require you to undertake placements outside of your base placement where you are employed. Depending on the range of experiences your organisation can offer, you may be able to take additional placements within your employing organisation or you may need to undertake some in other organisations. For example, a large acute NHS hospital trust could offer a range of placements to adult and child field students but not community placements (unless it is an integrated NHS trust). For learning disability nursing, you will most likely need placements across a wide range of NHS and independent health, education and social care providers outside of your base placement. Most mental health trusts can provide a range of experiences but may link with an acute hospital NHS trust to offer you an opportunity to develop your adult physical health skills. Therefore, if you are required to undertake placements outside of your employing organisation, many of the sections in this chapter will be important in helping you to prepare for your travel to the placement, getting to know the placement, and common fears and anxieties.

# Pre-placement checklist

Before your first shift, ensure you have everything ready for the next day. This means you have less to worry about, which may help you get a better night's sleep. If possible, aim to leave earlier than you need to, to ensure that you get there on time. This allows for unforeseen problems with travel and will reduce your stress considerably. If you do run into travel problems, let the placement know.

Below is a checklist to help you ensure you are ready for your first day:

- Uniform or appropriate clean clothes (if uniform not required) – all prepared
- Name badge/ID card
- Work shoes – cleaned and worn in
- Pens (in different colours) and small notebook
- List of keywords and abbreviations relevant to your placement
- Key textbook so you can look things up if you need to
- Journey details to your placement and return home (train/bus times, car journey/walking directions), including the time last trains/buses run
- Watch/fob watch
- Hair accessories to ensure hair tied up and off your shoulders
- Jewellery removed (a plain wedding band and ear studs are usually allowed)
- Tube of hand cream (frequent handwashing plays havoc with your skin)
- Lip cream (wards can be very drying)
- Food and drink to last the shift
- Practice Assessment Document and Ongoing Achievement Record
- Childcare back-up plans

## Chapter summary

This chapter has looked at the preparation you need to undertake prior to each placement, starting from the allocation process, and looked at the different types of placements you may be allocated to. Taking time to research the organisations you will be placed at will help you to plan your travel and help you to become familiar with the values of each organisation and the range of learning experiences available to you. Reading around the specialisms the placement offers will increase your confidence in understanding new terminology and ensure that the care you give is based on best evidence. This shows the staff on your placement that you have prepared and are interested in learning, which will reap benefits as they will invest more time in students who are engaged with the learning process. Nerves are normal before each placement, but good preparation will help reduce the nerves and ensure that you are in the best position to make the most of your time there.

# Activities: brief outline answers

## Activity 2.1 Critical thinking (p25)

You might suggest the following:

Make an appointment to talk to his personal tutor to discuss the different types of placements he will be undertaking on his programme and how the learning from them can be applied to his future career plans.

Look at the NMC standards and proficiencies – the aim of a pre-registration nursing programme is to develop a well-rounded registered nurse who meets these standards and has a range of knowledge and skills. Specialisation occurs after qualifying, and he can still apply for a post in a drug and alcohol recovery team (DART) or substance misuse service on qualifying.

He could ask the university if they allow students to request a specific type of placement in their final year.

He can still explore this area through some of his assignments.

## Activity 2.3 Critical thinking (p29)

Search the library to see if there is a key text on the speciality, or the NICE website (**www.nice.org.uk**) for guidelines related to the speciality.

The NHS website (**www.nhs.uk/conditions/**) covers a wide range of conditions for all ages and common mental health disorders.

Look at charity websites that focus on specific conditions (e.g. Diabetes UK, Mind, British Heart Foundation, Cancer Research UK).

Become familiar with common medical and Latin abbreviations used by doctors in prescriptions and notes (see **https://bnf.nice.org.uk/about/abbreviations-and-symbols.html**).

## Activity 2.4   Critical thinking (p30)

Possible answers you may have given are:

- Arrange to visit the ward to meet with a member of staff to talk through some of the questions you have; a face-to-face chat, even if brief, can help answer questions and allay fears.
- Leave your contact details so the placement can contact you later.
- Talk to the named person from the university linked to your placement or your personal tutor.

The problem with a response such as this is that not knowing anything about your placement until you get there limits how much preparation you can do beforehand. It is also difficult to plan your personal life, such as arranging childcare or organising paid work commitments, if you do not know what your shifts are.

## Activity 2.7   Research (p34)

The types of sessions you may have identified are likely to include some or all of the following:

- fire safety awareness training;
- key health and safety policies;
- manual handling training;
- infection control and hand hygiene;
- information governance and data handling;
- basic life support;
- equality, diversity and human rights;
- patient and student safety;
- safeguarding adults and children;
- conflict resolution/managing aggression; and
- Prevent training.

## Further reading

**Barr, O. and Gates, B.** (2018) *Oxford Handbook of Learning and Intellectual Disability Nursing,* 2nd edn. Oxford: Oxford University Press.

**Elcock, K., Everett, F., Newcombe, P. and Wright, W.** (2018) *Essentials of Nursing Adults.* London: SAGE.

**Price, J. and McAlinden, O.** (2017) *Essentials of Nursing Children and Young People.* London: SAGE.

**Wright, K.M. and McKeown, M.** (2018) *Essentials of Mental Health Nursing.* London: SAGE.

Each of the above books focuses on a specific field of nursing. Owning a book that covers your field of practice is essential in helping you prepare for the different types of placements you will experience.

## Useful websites

The Queen's Nursing Institute

**www.qni.org.uk/nursing-in-the-community/work-of-community-nurses/**

Describes the work of a wide range of different community nurses across all fields.

Student nurse video blogs

**www.youtube.com/playlist?list=PLoeGpqILd2rjCIqDG33JYsVMw1PHhSK5E**

A series of videos by student nurses that look at studying, placements and work-life balance.

Health Careers: Your First Placement

**www.healthcareers.nhs.uk/career-planning/study-and-training/considering-or-university/
support-university/your-first-placement**

Aimed at healthcare students, this web page has some valuable tips for first and future placements.

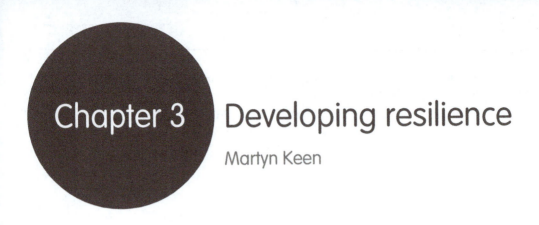

# Chapter 3  Developing resilience

Martyn Keen

---

### NMC Standards of Proficiency for Registered Nurses

This chapter will address the following platforms and proficiencies:

**Platform 1: Being an accountable professional**

Registered nurses act in the best interests of people, putting them first and providing nursing care that is person-centred, safe and compassionate. They act professionally at all times and use their knowledge and experience to make evidence-based decisions about care. They communicate effectively, are role models for others, and are accountable for their actions. Registered nurses continually reflect on their practice and keep abreast of new and emerging developments in nursing, health and care.

At the point of registration, the registered nurse will be able to:

1.1  understand and act in accordance with *The Code: Professional Standards of Practice and Behaviour for Nurses, Midwives and Nursing Associates*, and fulfil all registration requirements.

1.3  understand and apply the principles of courage, transparency and the professional duty of candour, recognising and reporting any situations, behaviours or errors that could result in poor care outcomes.

1.5  understand the demands of professional practice and demonstrate how to recognise signs of vulnerability in themselves or their colleagues and the action required to minimise risks to health.

1.6  understand the professional responsibility to adopt a healthy lifestyle to maintain the level of personal fitness and wellbeing required to meet people's needs for mental and physical care.

1.10 demonstrate resilience and emotional intelligence and be capable of explaining the rationale that influences their judgements and decisions in routine, complex and challenging situations.

## Chapter aims

After reading this chapter, you will be able to:

- define the holistic concept of resilience;
- appreciate the importance of being resilient in nursing and how it relates to our professional responsibilities;
- identify common sources of adversity for nursing students at university and consider how resilience can be used to effectively manage these; and
- identify key skills in strengthening your own resilience and how to have a positive influence on others.

*The oak fought the wind and was broken, the willow bent when it must and survived.*

(Robert Jorden)

# Introduction

In 1940, the UK was engaged in one of the largest military conflicts the world had experienced. During May of that year, the British and French armies had been over-run by German forces and were facing imminent defeat. The entire Allied forces were cornered in a town on the French coast called Dunkirk. What happened next has been seen by historians as one of the most significant examples of overcoming adversity and resilience the world has ever seen. In the face of insurmountable odds, Prime Minister Winston Churchill led on a plan to rescue as many of the 350,000 men at Dunkirk as possible, though the realistic expectation was that only a fraction would actually be saved. This tested the resilience and skills of a nation; the rest, as they say, is history. The final number rescued was over 330,000.

What has this story got to do with nursing? Well, in healthcare, the pressures and pace of change worldwide has meant nurses face increasing levels of adversity that require creative problem-solving driven by a strong emphasis on the concepts of courage, resilience and a belief that situations can change. Our business is about people too, so in a way we experience our own mini Dunkirks every day, and how we develop and strengthen our abilities in overcoming complex problems is an essential requirement in healthcare settings today if we are to deliver the highest quality of care for our patients.

So, let's journey together through this chapter to discover what we truly mean by the concept of resilience and how it forms an essential component in our professional tool-box as nurses.

# What is resilience?

Nelson Mandela famously said that 'The greatest glory in living lies not in never falling but rising every time we fall'. This beautifully highlights the importance in focusing not just on the adversities we face, but more on how we deal with them, and links appropriately with suggested general definitions of resilience. The term derives from the Latin *resiliere*, meaning 'to rebound' or 'to leap back'. Resilience is therefore viewed as a person's ability to adjust and adapt positively to complex situations and misfortune, with the aim of overcoming the difficulties experienced and growing stronger in the process (Jackson et al., 2007; Thomas and Asselin, 2017). This has also been termed as the process of 'bouncing back' from hard times, a respectful nod to the origins of the word. This concept was adopted into common culture in the UK when, in 2004, Ian Dowie, the then-manager of Crystal Palace Football Club, termed the phrase 'bouncebackability' to describe his team when they made a remarkable improvement that season. This term was so popular that it was added to the *Oxford English Dictionary* and even used in parliament as a way of describing resilience. Activity 3.1 is a simple reflective exercise to help you focus on identifying your own natural resilience skills.

## Activity 3.1   Reflection

Think back to the last time you faced an event that made you feel stressed. Can you recognise what you did to overcome this feeling?

Think about what you did and whether it helped.

Were other people involved in helping you with this event? If so, how did they help?

Write out a list of all the actions you or others used to help you through this event.

*As this activity is based on your own experiences, there is no outline answer at the end of the chapter.*

As we go further through this chapter, you can compare your answers above to the suggested activities we will cover. This will help you identify your natural resilience skills and confirm they are present in all of us.

## A closer look

Resilience is a concept of increasing interest worldwide and is being researched to determine the exact components that people adopt. A common debated view is that resilience is all about our character, with some people being more resilient to hardship due to inherent characteristics whereas others may not be. While elements of how we grow as individuals and form the characteristics of our personalities can have an impact on resilience, this is not the only determinant. Psychological studies over the last 40 years have identified that multiple holistic factors are at play in how we form and develop our skills of resilience from an early age, with agreement that this is a central part of human survivability (Taylor, 2019). The good news, therefore, is that we all have it, and we can nurture and grow our skills in resilience, and consequently strengthen our abilities to manage adversity. Later on in the chapter, we will explore this further and consider what we, as nurses, can do to increase our abilities to be resilient. However, to provide further clarity, let's turn first to specifically how resilience relates to nursing and why it is an essential element of our professional identity.

# Resilience and its importance in nursing

From its inception in 1948, the NHS has been an example of how a large organisation has had to cope and adapt to change in order to continue to meet the demand of a healthcare service free at the point of delivery. Nurses are the largest employed profession in the health service and seen as the very backbone of care. However, in recent times, the UK health system has been faced with significant challenges, including increasing population size with a higher life expectancy, increasing use of modern technology and care advancements, and the ever-present issues of infinite demand with finite resources. It has been reported that the current adversities faced by the NHS are some of the most significant issues ever faced in healthcare (NHS, 2019b).

With this in mind, the impact on modern-day nursing is exceptional and concerning. The Health and Safety Executive reported that in 2017–2018, 1.4 million people in the UK suffered work-based illnesses; the largest recorded illness group (44 per cent) was for stress-related, depression and anxiety issues (HSE, 2018). Sadly, public-sector workers were most at risk, with education, healthcare and social work seen as the three highest-risk groups, respectively. The most common reported causes were workload pressures, lack of support and organisational change. While this is worrying, remember that resilience is concerned with how we deal with pressures, not the pressures themselves. Therefore, in order to approach these issues differently, we first have to recognise in ourselves and in others the signs that situations require further consideration. So, we will now turn to explore stress and two concepts important in nursing: workplace burnout and compassion fatigue.

# Stress

Stress is a term used for a collection of psychological and physiological responses to a perceived threat from a situation or life event. Everyone has this natural response, though it is highly individual and can be determined by our environments and our own personalities. In essence, stress can be a positive experience as it heightens our awareness of threats and provides us with the ability to respond. Problems arise, however, when we perceive that the events are unmanageable or out of our control. Chronic feelings of unmanaged stress can result in negative experiences, such as anxiety issues and links to increased physical health issues (Mental Health Foundation, 2019).

Table 3.1 lists common signs of stress, which can be divided into different groups.

| Holistic elements | Signs of stress |
|---|---|
| Physical | Headaches |
| | Muscle tension or unexplained pain |
| | Experiencing dizziness |
| | Sleep problems |
| | Persistent tiredness |
| | Eating too much or too little |
| Emotional | Feeling overwhelmed |
| | Increased irritability |
| | Anxiety or unexplained feelings of fear |
| | Reduced self-esteem |
| Mental | Constant worrying |
| | Racing thought patterns |
| | Concentration difficulties |
| | Difficulties in making decisions |
| Behavioural | Avoidance of people and situations |
| | Snapping at others |
| | Increases in the use of substances (e.g. alcohol) |
| Social | Relationship difficulties with colleagues and at home |
| | Social withdrawal |
| | Impacts on sickness and lost productivity |

*Table 3.1*   Common signs of stress

*Source:* Adapted from NHS (2019a)

The experiences in the workplace of chronic unmanaged stress has led to increased interest in exploring the concept known as burnout.

# Burnout

Burnout was first termed in 1974 when a study into healthcare workers demonstrated certain experiences when under occupational-related stress. These included persistent exhaustion, physical symptoms, thinking problems and emotional outbursts. Due to the increase in occupational health issues since this time, research into this phenomenon has grown (Freudenberger, 1974). The World Health Organization has included burnout as part of the international classification of diseases, defining it as an occupational syndrome identified by a collection of signs present caused by unmanaged and chronic work-related stress (WHO, 2018). They have highlighted it as one of the main concerns for work-related health issues in the world, which is typified by three dimensions:

1. feelings of energy depletion or exhaustion;
2. increased mental distance from one's job and/or feelings of negativism or cynicism; and
3. reduced professional efficacy.

It is noted that this definition is specifically defined for workplace-related problems, and as such the term 'burnout' is seen very much as a work-based syndrome that relates to all occupational environments. However, a concept that is perhaps more related to healthcare is another phenomenon: compassion fatigue.

## Compassion fatigue

Compassion fatigue particularly affects those individuals with caregiving responsibilities and is defined as an intense preoccupation of the distress of others in the absence of caring for oneself. Left to continue, a person can experience extreme signs of apathy, preoccupied thinking, altered behaviour and emotional burnout. Ultimately, this can lead to secondary post-trauma conditions that can have damaging psychological implications. The difference here from burnout is that the person's trauma is related to their preoccupation on the distress of another as the cause, rather than purely work-related factors (Gallagher, 2013). Again, early recognition is key here, with the involvement of quality support in practice and clinical supervision. Consider Margaret's case study below and complete Activity 3.2. This will help you to identify the different types of stress, as well as consider potential responses to working with people in distress.

### Case study: Margaret

Margaret is a second-year children's nursing student who is currently placed in a paediatric palliative care environment as part of a seven-week placement. She is a committed and caring person and has been focused on caring for her patients while completing her latest academic assignment. Margaret highlighted to her friend that she has been having trouble sleeping over the last two nights and has noted a reduction in appetite. Yesterday she said she felt light-headed on her way home from work. Finally, she admits that the combination of caring for children who are dying, which she has not experienced before, and her studies is making her feel overwhelmed at times. However, she continues going to work and is completing her assignment.

## Activity 3.2   Critical thinking

Looking at Margaret's experience, would you say she is stressed, burnt out or suffering from compassion fatigue?

What evidence do you see that would support your choice?

If you were Margaret's friend, what would you say to her?

*An outline answer to this activity is given at the end of the chapter.*

The causes related to these phenomena will always be issues we may have to face at times, but by building up our skills of how we face these adversities it is perfectly possible to not only overcome them but become stronger professionally and personally in the process. It's useful at this point to consider in further detail what resilient people in nursing look like.

Well, in truth, they look like you and me, people who already have comprehensive strategies for dealing with complex nursing issues; though these are not exclusive to nursing, they are inspirational and serve as an excellent reference for us all to learn from. **Social psychology** suggests that one of the most powerful ways of improving ourselves is learning through the actions and experiences of others. To consider this further, complete Activity 3.3.

## Activity 3.3   Reflection

Think of one inspirational individual, either in popular culture or personally to you, that overcame significant adversity, and consider the following questions:

- What do you admire in them the most?
- Write down three of the most important characteristics that the individual displayed during this event that you think had the most positive impact on overcoming adversity.
- Look at these three characteristics and consider why these are particularly important to you.
- What did you learn from this person's example that may impact on your ability to be inspirational when facing adversity?

*As this activity is based on your own observation, there is no outline answer at the end of the chapter.*

# Student adversity issues

Choosing to become a student in higher education, whether for the first time, coming straight from school or choosing a new direction later in life, can be an exciting and life-changing event. The opportunity to learn new topics, experience new environments and meet new people can have a significant impact on how we grow and develop in life. However, university life can bring other experiences that we need to be mindful of, which, if unmanaged, can impair progression and impact on our well-being. This section will consider some of these pitfalls and offer simple yet effective strategies in overcoming adversities to keep you on track to reaching your maximum potential. The examples here are based on real student experiences and offer insight into what to look out for and how to help yourself and others.

You will discover during your education that holistic approaches to care are seen as a cornerstone of nursing. Holism recognises that the individual as a whole is greater than the sum of its parts. Our experiences are made up of a combination of social, environmental, psychological, biological and spiritual elements, but holism understands these are interdependent and each part is closely related (Brooker and Waugh, 2013). There are more areas if you subdivide down, though the content for each section is entirely unique to the person (Figure 3.1).

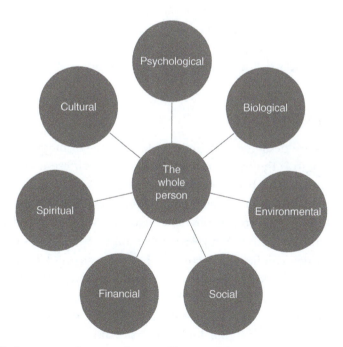

*Figure 3.1* Holistic approach to understanding people

The same principles apply to ourselves when we look at the sources and solutions to stress. With this in mind, it's helpful to look at the different types of potential stressors that you may face during your time at university. Let's look at some of the common issues that students have reported; while there are many, these are some of the popular issues raised.

# Financial issues

In my discussions with students from a diverse collection of backgrounds and cultures, a number of themed issues were identified as key areas for stress. As we have already seen, stress in itself is not necessarily a negative experience, though the situations described here were seen as having the potential to cause adverse reactions while at university.

A common reported area of social/environmental concern to students was the significant and constant pressure of balancing financial issues at university. People understand that financial sacrifices are expected when coming to university, though the full impact of this can hit students at any time, and can be a clear cause of distress and altered well-being:

> *I didn't realise the full extent of balancing my finances, particularly when on placement, writing assignments and having to maintain a part-time income at the same time. It's really stressful.*

In these circumstances, it is important to talk through these issues with your family and the university, which will have financial support services specifically to help students. The student union is also helpful in navigating the support available, as well as your personal tutor, who can assist in looking at work-life balance.

# Living away from home

Socially, universities are designed to bring people together from a wide range of communities. A main strength is the opportunity to understand different cultures, experiences and viewpoints. However, in bringing people together, there is the inevitable potential for increased conflict. For students, living away from home for the first time with friends sounds like a blast, but when your room-mate leaves dirty dishes in the sink and eats the cheesecake you were saving, then tempers can get a little fraught! It's uncommon, but in extreme situations open conflict can occur, which leads to stressful living and a breakdown in relationships. This is a good example of a link across the holistic elements, as stressful living conditions can lead to psychological problems and poor sleep, as well as affecting study, among other problems. Similarly, renting and problems with challenging landlords is another common issue. In fact, our local university support service highlighted accommodation problems as the most common reason students sought support:

> *I thought it would be fun living in halls with people of my own age. But when you have to get up for an early shift and the student upstairs is playing loud music all night, I could scream!*

The first suggestion here is to approach the person and discuss your concerns. It is often the case that individuals don't know they are being annoying, and easy compromises are achieved simply through talking. Allowing the situation to drag on will only lead to things worsening. University-provided residences have support services attached and will have processes of mediation for complaints if things become challenging. As a last resort, it may be that a change in living accommodation is the only solution, which, while stressful, can have a dramatic improvement on the situation. For private renting, again engage with your landlord about concerns you have. Should you need legal advice, services such as Citizens Advice and indeed the student union may be able to guide you further.

Students who remain at home can also feel isolated because their family do not understand the demands of a nursing course, as well as why shifts cannot always accommodate family events and holidays are fixed. These students also have less contact with their peers when off-duty, losing access to an important support network.

## Impact on own mental health

Of course, the nursing programme itself will bring its own issues that may affect our ability to successfully progress. As discussed in earlier chapters, nursing as a professional-based vocation holds expectations on how we conduct ourselves professionally, the knowledge we need to care safely, and our approaches to people in distress, and it is no secret that the nature of nursing can be stressful.

As students, this could be the first time you have been exposed to such high professional expectations. These, alongside academic learning and clinical care, will naturally impact on your holistic well-being, particularly the internal aspects of being human and your emotional and psychological responses. Our mental well-being is a crucial component in caring for others. 'If we struggle to manage ourselves, how can we help others?' is a well-known phrase. A YouGov (2016) poll identified that 27 per cent of university students reported experiencing a mental health problem. Women were reported to be at higher risk, though caution needs to be paid here as men are generally less likely to report health issues. Of significance were the rates of mental health issues in the LGBTQ communities (45 per cent). Universities pride themselves on inclusion and diversity, though the facts remain that LGBTQ populations face additional struggles and require tailored support services. Seeking out LGBTQ-centric student groups can be a great source of support and advice, so do consider seeking these out at your chosen institution.

The most common conditions reported were depression and anxiety, followed by eating disorders. In my professional experience, these are common issues reported by students. However, it is worth noting that the prevalence of other serious mental health-related conditions are regularly experienced in university populations too. Further examples can include psychotic-related experiences, behavioural/developmental conditions, learning disabilities and personality issues. Life events are a natural occurrence in all our lives, though events such as relationship break-ups and bereavement are difficult at any time. Couple this with a stressful course such as nursing, though, and it can make the ability to manage situations even more challenging. There are other secondary social issues that are worth mentioning, including substance use conditions and gambling, which can either cause or maintain problems too. Sadly, examples of traumatic social events, such as homelessness and domestic violence, can also arise and require urgent action; the university can support you through this and assist you in finding the courage to face situations such as these, which should not happen to anyone.

## Students with dyslexia

University attendance can also help in identifying issues you may not have been aware of. Language-based learning disabilities such as dyslexia affect 10 per cent of the population in the UK, and dyslexia is officially identified as a disability in the Equality Act 2010 as it affects a person's ability to achieve their full potential. Some students fear academic work due to past poor performance at school, but university is not school, and understanding how you learn is an important part of being successful. If you believe you may be dyslexic, it is important to raise this with your personal tutor. Dyslexic assessments are available and can explain difficulties that you may have had all your life for the first time. Even better, if diagnosed, academic support plans and even funding options can be accessed that can give you the improved learning resources you need in order to succeed. This is explored further in Chapter 8.

# Support available for students

The diverse support services at universities are important in helping students with a range of issues. Each organisation has its own dedicated student well-being services, which include practical help and advice, counselling, and advocacy for a range of issues, including disability support and mental health. If you have a pre-existing health issue, it is important to declare this at application. The nursing workforce needs to represent the communities it serves, and having staff with lived experience of physical, mental, developmental and/or social issues is seen as a strength, and people are actively encouraged to join; indeed, this is often the reason people choose nursing. However, in order to minimise the impact of any existing issue, working with the support services and education staff from an early stage is hugely beneficial. Once disclosed, you will have access to personalised support plans, named mental health or disability advisors, and support in ensuring learning is tailored to your needs. A strong relationship with your allocated personal tutor can help identify issues early and ensure support is put in place quickly and in confidence in order to support your performance. Finally, never underestimate the love and support of your family and friends, including your peers at university. The tough days you will have at times are better experienced with trusted people than experienced alone. Your student peer group in particular knows the reality of being a student and is an important source of support.

I have personally seen a wide range of strong and resourceful students who have successfully managed their health and social issues in partnership with support services at university. Watching these magnificent people grow and transform into professional nurses has been a humbling and inspiring experience. I think this teaches us that we all hold an ability to overcome our own Dunkirks, and our experiences – good or bad – can enrich our lives if we work at them, though early identification and making choices of who we get support from is key. To explore how this may work, let's look at another case study and then complete Activity 3.4.

## Case study: Ade

Ade is a 37-year-old lady of Nigerian heritage who came to live in the UK five years ago with her family, husband Michael and 15-year-old son Daniel, who has recently been diagnosed with dyslexia. Ade has always worked in the caring profession, and after a period working in nursing home care decided to undertake a degree in pre-registration nursing. The university is a two-hour journey from home. At first, university life was exciting, and Ade met new people, achieved well in her first assignments and liked being in her first mental health placement. She also worked part-time in her local care home to support the family's finances at weekends. However, nine months in, while in her third placement, an acute inpatient service, Ade had a challenging experience. The travel was long and shift work was frequent. Her practice supervisor appeared overworked and their relationship was strained at times. Towards the end, Ade worked closely with a patient who sadly died by suicide, but was unable to discuss this with anyone, only being told, 'It's part of the job'. Following this, Ade struggled to concentrate and did not hand in her final Year 1 essay. She felt she had failed herself and her family and began experiencing anxiety and sleep problems. Two years previously, Ade was diagnosed with depression and worried the feelings had returned. Ade feared that if she disclosed her situation to the university, she would be dismissed, which would lead to feelings of shame.

## Activity 3.4   Critical thinking

What were the events that led to Ade feeling distressed? Consider all the holistic elements to guide you.

Why do you think Ade is frightened of disclosing her feelings to the university?

If you were Ade's best friend, what would be your advice, and why?

*An outline answer to this activity is given at the end of the chapter.*

# How can we strengthen our resilience?

We introduced resilience earlier in the chapter and established how important this is for nurses, so let's now look at some practical strategies that we can use in order to strengthen our abilities in managing adversity.

The ancient Greek philosopher Socrates once remarked, 'To find yourself, think for yourself'. In essence, this suggests that a truer appreciation of ourselves leads to a clearer understanding of how you react to situations and the impact you have on the world around you. Professional self-awareness is integral within our professional regulations. *The Code* (NMC, 2018a) highlights the importance of professional and personal reflection, as well as how this influences decision-making and our relationships with others and how we look after ourselves. A stronger emphasis on self-resilience is also expected to be included in all new curricula as part of the revised education standards for pre-registration nursing (NMC, 2018e), so it's clear to see how importantly this is viewed.

The purpose of resilience has two main functions: first, strategies to protect us from stressful events and build our tolerance; and second, skills to enhance our abilities in bouncing back from adversity in order to not only return to our acceptable level of functioning, but become stronger through learnt experience. With this in mind, let's explore some practical approaches that are helpful in addressing both these aims.

## Breathing

An effective short-term technique to manage stress is to breathe. It sounds simple and something we all do all the time; however, breathing is one of the few semi-autonomic physical functions we can have some control over and is used in everything from pregnancy to public speaking. Adversity can lead to feelings of anxiety and panic, yet by consciously stopping, focusing on our breathing style and completing simple exercises, the impact on the initial distress can be dramatic. Box 3.1 offers a simple technique supported by the NHS (2018b).

---

### Box 3.1  Breathing technique for relaxation and reducing stress

You will get the most benefit if you do it regularly, as part of your daily routine.

You can do it standing up, sitting in a chair that supports your back, or lying on a bed or yoga mat on the floor.

Make yourself as comfortable as you can. If you can, loosen any clothes that restrict your breathing.

---

If you're lying down, place your arms a little bit away from your sides, with the palms up. Let your legs be straight, or bend your knees so your feet are flat on the floor.

If you're sitting, place your arms on the chair arms.

If you're sitting or standing, place both feet flat on the ground. Whatever position you're in, place your feet roughly hip-width apart.

- Let your breath flow as deep down into your belly as is comfortable, without forcing it.
- Try breathing in through your nose and out through your mouth.
- Breathe in gently and regularly. Some people find it helpful to count steadily from one to five. You may not be able to reach five at first.
- Then, without pausing or holding your breath, let it flow out gently, counting from one to five again, if you find this helpful.
- Keep doing this for three to five minutes.

*Source*: NHS (2018b)

This exercise can be done anywhere at any time, and is a simple strategy to regain control back over the situation. Try this out and check to see whether your emotions change. The more you practise, the more it can become part of your resilience toolbox. Technology also assists, with a number of useful phone applications, such as Happy Not Perfect, or many smartwatches that have built-in relaxation tools. Try it out – you may surprise yourself.

# Emotional intelligence and mindfulness

Franklin D. Roosevelt famously said, 'We have nothing to fear but fear itself', a powerful and insightful suggestion that suggests we fear more the thought of being frightened by situations rather than the situation itself. Nursing is a complex and demanding profession that has the ability to cause emotional distress through the care of some of the most vulnerable people in our society. We have already seen that, left unchecked, this can have a detrimental impact on our well-being and on the quality of care we deliver. High levels of unmanaged emotion and poor management of stress were highlighted in the Francis Report as influential in the tragic outcomes seen there (Francis, 2013). However, key in becoming a resilient nurse is a conscious understanding of our own emotions and how they influence our health and our wider world. Two approaches to address this are emotional intelligence and mindfulness. We will now explore each in turn to understand the relevance for us as nurses.

# Emotional intelligence

*The Code* (NMC, 2018a) is clear that a strong sense of professional self-awareness is a professional expectation that guides nurses to develop robust strategies in regularly reflecting back on their professional behaviour and emotions with a view of managing their own well-being. After all, in order to deliver compassionate and highly skilled care for others, there is a need to first be caring towards ourselves; addressing our own needs is therefore paramount to successful nursing. So, how do we do this?

Emotional intelligence was developed by Goleman (1999) as a strategy to improve our relations with ourselves and others. The process begins when we are young and involves developing competence in a number of skills, including these main areas:

- *self-awareness*: awareness of your own individuality;
- *empathy*: an appreciation of another's feelings;
- *congruence*: being appropriate in a given situation;
- *honesty*: the personal quality of truthfulness.

Creating an intelligent awareness of ourselves and others provides us with insight into situations, and therefore a clearer view on the correct approaches to use. Take a look at the following case study, which explains how.

## Case study: Hafez

Hafez, a final-year adult nurse, is working with Gary, a 50-year-old gentleman who is recovering from a myocardial infarction in a cardiac unit. Gary is in pain, which is being managed, though he is obviously still distressed. He has never been in hospital before and owns his own construction business and lives alone. This morning, he shouted at Hafez during the morning drug round and called him 'useless' for not getting him well quick enough. Hafez is upset by this and discusses the incident with his practice supervisor.

Through supervision, Hafez and his practice supervisor identify that it is unacceptable for nurses to be shouted at by patients. However, using empathy, they considered why Gary may be emotional; he was perhaps first frightened by the diagnosis, the environment and the potential prognosis. He is an independent man with responsibilities but little in the way of a social support network. A fear of losing his business and managing a serious health concern on his own is a daunting concept. They acknowledged that Gary was also in pain, which had an impact on his emotions. Through using professional awareness, Hafez was able to see he had not done anything wrong. The incident was not personal and was perhaps more linked with Gary's obvious sources of distress. This changed Hafez's view, and consequently his emotion, to one of how difficult it must be for Gary. They agreed to speak to Gary first to reinforce that shouting at staff is not acceptable but also to explore his sources of distress. Gary was apologetic and confirmed he didn't understand the diagnosis and was worried about the future and his business, which made him frustrated and frightened. This opened up further discussions on helping Gary understand his illness and plans for the future, including lifestyle changes he could make.

You can see from this case study the components of emotional intelligence in operation. Hafez was correct in controlling his emotions and seeking supervision to help him make sense of the situation. They correctly assisted Gary in an honest conversation on the understanding of professional boundaries involved in care. Through using empathy and self-awareness techniques, they were able to discover a more informed insight, leading to new care directions, in this case health education and social planning. If this had just been left, it is likely the working relationship would have been impaired and other holistic aspects of Gary's care missed.

## Mindfulness

Mindfulness is seen as a concept in directing us to know and be kind to ourselves. Sometimes our worst enemy is our self and the unfair pressure we place on our expectations and achievements. These are often driven externally by social pressure and peer influence; in a world of social media and fake news, this has become increasingly more difficult to manage. Mindfulness is useful in all walks of life, being used not only in healthcare, but in areas such as school, being applicable for people of all ages and cultures. It is defined broadly as:

*Purposefully paying attention to the present moment in a non-judgemental way. It consists in observing what is happening moment by moment in one's internal (thoughts, motives, emotions, bodily sensations) and external world without judging it.*

(Peña-Sarrionandia et al., 2015, p4)

The historic origins are seen in a range of spiritual belief systems, though principally Buddhism. It has now gathered in popularity within the wider community, being widely researched and supported as a valid approach to managing our psychological well-being.

So, it is a process of listening to our thoughts, exploring our feelings and noticing how our body reacts in a given moment. We could say we are talking to ourselves all the time, but mindfulness encourages us to listen and make sense of it in order to move forward. It sounds easy, but factor in our busy lives, the adversities, fatigue and many other experiences, and our ability to concentrate back on ourselves becomes less of a feature, and often we can get lost in the bigger picture.

Consider these two responses from a student who has received a grade for their latest piece of academic work:

> *I only got a B and wanted an A. This took a lot of work and I'm exhausted and frustrated. I feel useless.*

This is a common response we take towards disappointment, mostly driven by our emotion and an automatic ability to be self-critical. You can see how the person refers to their emotions, self-opinion and physical state, but doesn't acknowledge the present rational elements of the situation. An alternative view may be:

> *I am disappointed; though I passed this assignment with a good mark, it will be important to learn what can be developed in my writing in order to improve my future grades. I think I need to look after myself better as this work has made me feel drained.*

This alternative response still contains reference to the elements mentioned above but takes a more rational-based view of the present, with future plans to address the issues present.

## Differing minds

To get further clarity on how our minds operate, one mindfulness theory suggests that we have three minds: the emotional mind, the logical mind and the wise mind. All can operate within us, but at times, or due to our character, one can dominate the others:

- *Emotional mind*: Formed from our subcortical or primitive brain centres. Characterised by a domination of emotive-led thinking and behaviour, where we present as irritable and hot-headed.
- *Logical mind*: Driven by the frontal cortex, which provides the logical and problem-solving element of our brain's functioning. When this is a dominant feature, people present as logical and emotionally detached.
- *Wise mind*: A point in thinking where the two integrate in order to create balance. A person here will present as calm but emotionally aware of themselves and others. This is more conducive for compassionate approaches but requires more conscious attention in refining it further.

(Kabat-Zinn, 2013, cited in Gault et al., 2017, p47)

Now consider these three areas in relation to your own experiences in Activity 3.5.

## Activity 3.5   Critical thinking

First, use your observing eye to ascertain how you are reacting to university, work and personal demands. Are there different reactions at different times? See if you can think of a time when each of the three minds was dominant:

- *Emotional mind*: Are you overusing your emotional mind? Do you focus on completing tasks despite the impact on others or on your own well-being? Do you find it difficult to move away from task orientation and think about the implications of your actions? During this example, how did you feel before, during and afterwards?
- *Logical mind*: Can you think of a time when tasks were focused with a view of rationalising your behaviour to ignore the emotions of others and detach yourself from the experience?
- *Wise mind*: Consider a time when you were able to be both compassionate yet focused and logical in your actions at the same time.

(adapted from Gault et al., 2017, p47)

*As this activity is based on your own observation, there is no outline answer at the end of the chapter.*

The following points will help you to analyse situations and employ a more balanced approach:

- What am I thinking?
- What are my priorities and how are my current feelings impacting on these?
- What is the most important priority from the list, and why?
- What might be the worst possible outcome?
- What do I need to do to avoid the worst possible outcome?
- Which tasks are the most important to adopt now to prevent the worst possible outcome?

With a wise mind, we accept who we are, fallible and not superhuman. The response you make may not be the most ideal for all concerned, but it is considered, actions are prioritised, and the emotions of others and yourself are compassionately thought about. Try this third way the next time you face a challenging event and see if it alters the decisions and actions you take.

As humans, we are complex social beings that require a range of activities to improve and maintain our mental and physical health. Here are five steps for helping us make simple changes to our lifestyles:

1. connect with others;
2. be active;
3. keep learning;
4. give to others; and
5. be mindful.

(NHS, 2018a)

Now begin Activity 3.6. This will guide you in considering mindfulness-related choices that can have a positive impact on your well-being right now.

## Activity 3.6   Reflection

Look at the NHS Moodzone web page *5 Steps to Mental Wellbeing* (NHS, 2018a), which describes these steps in more detail, with additional links with further advice.

Reflect on which ones you could implement now to improve your mental well-being.

*As this activity is based on your own observation, there is no outline answer at the end of the chapter.*

With regard to step 2, the NHS web page *Get Active for Mental Wellbeing* (NHS, 2018c) suggests that adults aged over 19 years should aim for at least 150 minutes of moderate intensive aerobic activity a week. This could include regular walking, cycling or organised health classes. A well-recognised phone application, Couch to 5K, contains a steady and motivating audio and visual package to help people start running, and is worth considering. Of course, if you are concerned about your ability to conduct physical activity, it is important to consult your GP beforehand.

## Chapter summary

We hope you enjoyed this chapter; looking back, we discovered the importance of looking after ourselves as nurses, a rewarding but demanding profession, through channelling and strengthening our abilities to adopt resilience. We all face adversities at times in our lives, and nursing can bring us in contact with people experiencing some of the most vulnerable times in their lives. Learning to protect us from stress and burnout and discovering our own resilience toolbox will help us deliver more compassionate and meaningful care. From simple yet effective techniques of breathing and being active to more detailed approaches such as emotional intelligence and mindfulness, there are numerous ways we can find our own individual strategies for managing adversity. So, when we are faced with our Dunkirks, we will have the courage and fortitude to face them for the benefits of others, and importantly for our own well-being. As Jerry Springer used to say, 'Take care of yourselves and each other'.

# Activities: brief outline answers

## Activity 3.2    Critical thinking (p46)

It is likely Margaret is feeling signs of stress. The environment is one she is not used to, a common experience for students, which involves managing distress regularly. Although she is noticing signs, she is talking them through with a trusted friend and has only been experiencing these for a short while. Although she is feeling overwhelmed, she continues to go to work and is completing her studies and is therefore still functioning. If I was her friend, the therapeutic importance of listening to her may be all that is required. Offering social contact, whether a night in or going out socially, may also help. I may advise her to speak to her practice supervisor about her feelings and arrange regular supervision during the placement. If it persists, Margaret would need to inform her practice supervisor and her link lecturer from university or her personal tutor for further assistance in managing her workload and the emotional impact of the placement.

## Activity 3.4    Critical thinking (p51)

There are clear potential causes for Ade's distress: the rapid changing tasks attributed to nursing courses, such as exams, essays and numerous different practice placements, can take their toll. It's not uncommon to have a honeymoon period in the first year only later to go on and feel exhausted. Travel distances and shift work are common stressors, particularly for students with families. Traumatic clinical events, such as the loss of people we have cared for on placement, are also challenging. However, receiving initial debrief support, clinical supervision from your practice supervisor, personal tutor support and counselling (if required) are all formal systems that can help minimise the impact. Sadly, Ade did not receive any of this at the time and staff didn't pick up on the importance of this for her. It is hard work managing study and a family, and these strains can also impact on the stress. Additionally, trying to remain financially solvent can be hard, as is the case here.

The fear of disclosure is a common phenomenon, with common misconceptions that it is a weakness and will affect the person's record. It would be foolish to suggest discrimination does not exist but having challenges and illnesses does not impact on your nursing record, and indeed is a professional responsibility in looking after ourselves within *The Code*. Universities take support of students' needs seriously and confidentiality is assured, but this support can only be put in place if the issues are disclosed. Lastly, there may also be a cultural aspect for students to consider. Our cultural norms in managing adversity, the perceptions we hold of mental health and our relationships with our family can inhibit people from seeking help from others.

If I was Ade's friend, listening and being there are again important. Helping her make sense of the situation and looking at the options available can also be cathartic in helping Ade reach an informed choice on what will help. The option to raise this with the personal tutor will be important as this will open up access to further debriefing and help in planning academic support. Ade has had health problems in the past and encouraging her to consider seeking GP access and a referral to the university occupational health service can allow her needs to be professionally assessed for further intervention. Ultimately, it is an NMC requirement to look after our own health, which is seen as a strong professional attribute in nursing.

# Further reading

**Gault, I., Shapcott, J., Luthi, A. and Reid, G.** (2017) *Communication in Nursing and Healthcare.* London: SAGE.

Chapter 4, 'Enabling Positive Behaviour', provides further insight into clinical application of emotional intelligence as well as a focus on mindfulness and self-awareness.

**Sheridan, C.** (2016) *The Mindful Nurse: Using the Power of Mindfulness and Compassion to Help You Thrive in Your Work.* Galway: Rivertime Press.

A useful presentation of the importance of mindfulness in nursing, providing specific insight into its adaptation to the profession.

**Traynor, M.** (2017) *Critical Resilience for Nurses.* London: Routledge.

This text provides an interesting challenge to just adopting personal resilience, proposing that organisations are responsible in allowing nurses to practise resilience in their careers and are equally responsible.

## Useful websites

Citizens Advice

**www.citizensadvice.org.uk**

A national charity-based organisation offering independent advice on a wide range of social issues.

Nursing and Midwifery Standards

**www.nmc.org.uk/standards/**

This web page contains the education standards related to your programme, as well as *The Code* and additional guidance documents discussed in this chapter.

Royal College of Nursing: Healthy Workplace, Healthy You – Time and Space

**www.rcn.org.uk/healthy-workplace/healthy-you/time-and-space**

A series of short self-help mindfulness videos designed for nursing staff that focus on a specific part of the day. A useful resource for practical daily tips on managing stress and our well-being at work.

## Useful apps

Couch to 5K

**www.nhs.uk/live-well/exercise/couch-to-5k-week-by-week/**

This is an NHS-backed programme designed to help people improve their levels of activity and exercise. It consists of a nine-week course of focused goals supported with enjoyable podcasts, all accessed via an easy-to-use app.

Happy Not Perfect

**https://uk.happynotperfect.com**

Designed as a helpful companion app to help with mental well-being, stress management and sleep. Uses a motivational approach that helps us focus on positive psychology and mindfulness techniques for daily non-intrusive exercises designed to calm minds and improve our emotional welfare.

# Chapter 4

# Who can support you on placement?

Karen Chandler

(Continued)

others in the team including lay carers. They play an active and equal role in the interdisciplinary team, collaborating and communicating effectively with a range of colleagues.

At the point of registration, the registered nurse will be able to:

5.4 demonstrate an understanding of the roles, responsibilities and scope of practice of all members of the nursing and interdisciplinary team and how to make best use of the contributions of others involved in providing care.

## Chapter aims

After reading this chapter, you will be able to:

- explain how NMC standards inform the support systems in practice placement;
- identify the key roles to support students and learners in practice placements;
- identify other staff and resources that can provide support for you when on placement; and
- appreciate how research informs strategies for supporting students, supervisors and assessors in practice placement.

# Introduction

New situations can be stressful, whether that is starting a new school/college, moving away from home, starting university, or your first or subsequent placements on your nursing programme. You can feel a range of emotions, which can be scary; however, this chapter intends to help you recognise that these feelings are normal, and with support anxieties can be reduced. This support will come from a range of people, and in this chapter we will explore who these people might be and what roles and responsibilities they have to play in your learning on the nursing programme.

During your placement, you will be supported by staff – largely qualified nurses – who, as part of their professional code, are expected to facilitate your learning (NMC, 2018a). In 2018, the NMC published a new framework and set of standards that changed the way in which students are supported and assessed in practice, moving from **mentors and sign-off mentors** to practice supervisors and assessors.

# How do the standards inform the support systems in practice placement?

The *Standards of Proficiency* (NMC, 2018e) and *Standards for Student Supervision and Assessment* (SSSA) (NMC, 2018c) set out the structures of support that any student nurse, midwife, nursing associate or post-registration student can expect in practice. All universities, in partnership with placement providers, will have implemented these standards by September 2020. As a student, you will be supported by three new roles, described in the SSSA as practice supervisors (PS), practice assessors (PA) and academic assessors (AA). Practice supervisors are role models who will help to plan and supervise your learning experiences in practice, and you may have more than one of these on a placement. Practice assessors are responsible for assessing your progress and achievement of the NMC (2018c) proficiencies in practice. Academic assessors have oversight of your academic and practice progress. These three roles, working together, have been developed to support your progression through theory and practice. Let's look at each of these in a little more detail.

# Practice supervisors

The practice supervisor can be any health and social care registrant, who will:

- act as a role model in line with their professional code and their scope of practice to enable you to achieve the proficiencies;
- provide you with feedback on your progress, contributing to your achievement;
- appropriately raise and respond to matters relating to your conduct and competence; and
- have an understanding of the programme outcomes you are undertaking.

(NMC, 2018c, p6)

Their role emulates the supporting, supervising role of former mentors, but they are not making an overall judgement on your competency. They are, however, key to helping you understand the expectations of a professional. Each health and social care profession has professional expectations in relation to the conduct of their registrants, with commonalities across the professions. Your practice supervisor will therefore be able to provide you with feedback to help you understand the necessary skills, knowledge and attitudes expected of a professional.

## How will you benefit from the practice supervisor role?

The benefits can be summarised as follows:

- *Environment*: As a student, you will benefit from working with and learning from a range of people, and different professions, in the practice setting. For example, a newly qualified nurse/nursing associate is likely to understand some of the anxieties you are experiencing as a student on placement, and should be able to help you settle in and learn new skills and behaviours, whereas another health and social care professional, such as a physiotherapist or a social worker, will have had different learning experiences, and so an insight into these will be valuable to your own learning.

- *Supervision:* A practice supervisor will assist you in identifying learning opportunities, aiding you to enhance your skills and knowledge to develop as an autonomous practitioner, acting as a role model and sharing their expertise with you. They can also identify additional practice supervisors in conjunction with your practice assessor to help you develop more specific knowledge/skills.

- *Feedback:* A practice supervisor will provide you with feedback on your knowledge, clinical skills and professional competence to help you reflect and develop. They will also help inform your assessment by providing feedback to you and your practice assessor, identifying areas of achievement as well as areas for further development. Activity 4.1 asks you to consider what different practice supervisors can offer you.

## Activity 4.1   Critical thinking

You are about to commence your first placement on your programme. Consider who will be available to support you in your learning. Who might be identified as your practice supervisor(s), and how might they contribute to your learning?

*An outline answer to this activity is given at the end of the chapter.*

# Practice assessors

A practice assessor is:

- a registered nurse;
- appropriately prepared, maintaining their current knowledge and expertise; and
- knowledgeable about the proficiencies, programme outcomes and assessment process, with the interpersonal communication skills relevant to student learning/assessment.

They will:

- gather and coordinate feedback from practice supervisors and other relevant people;

- provide constructive feedback to facilitate development of others;
- conduct **objective, evidence-based assessment** based on feedback and observation; and
- reflect on their role and develop their own professional practice.

(NMC, 2018c, p9)

Your practice assessor will be assigned to you for a placement, or in exceptions for a series of placements across an assessed period or part of your programme. You should be informed who your practice assessor is from the beginning of the placement as they will be responsible for your overall assessment in practice.

## How will you benefit from the practice assessor role?

The benefits can be summarised as follows:

- *Environment*: They have a key role in overseeing your whole experience on a placement, working with practice supervisors to ensure that the learning opportunities enable you to meet programme requirements. They will also be involved in managing any concerns that arise regarding your performance and liaising with staff involved in supporting your learning.
- *Supervision*: The practice assessor will liaise with your practice supervisor(s) to monitor your progress and respond to queries they or you may have.
- *Assessment*: A key part of their role is to collate feedback on your performance and achievement from a number of sources in practice, although you should also be proactive in collating this evidence as you will know who you have worked with or where you have spent time. In order to undertake your assessment, they will have an understanding of your proficiencies and programme outcomes that you need to achieve, and will be able to conduct an objective, evidence-based assessment. They will use information gathered from your practice supervisor(s) and others you have worked with, alongside their own observations of your practice and the evidence you have gathered, in order to make an informed decision on whether you have demonstrated the appropriate knowledge, skills and attitudes in the proficiencies you are being assessed on. In addition, they have an important role in providing you with constructive feedback that will help you understand your strengths and areas you need to develop further. Should you not be making the expected progress, they will liaise with your academic assessor and develop an action plan, which will detail the actions needed to help you achieve the identified goals.

The NMC requires you to have a different practice assessor for each assessed period or part of your programme; therefore, if you find you have been allocated a practice assessor who you have had before, then you must inform the practice educator/ward manager or your university academic assessor/link lecturer to check this is not an issue.

# Academic assessors

The academic assessor will be a member of academic staff from your university, and – like the practice assessor – you cannot have the same academic assessor for two consecutive parts of your programme (NMC, 2018c).

Your academic assessor will:

- be a registered nurse;
- have an understanding of your learning and achievement in practice;
- collate and confirm your achievement of proficiencies and programme outcomes for each part in the academic environment;
- make and record objective, evidence-based decisions on conduct, proficiency and achievement, as well as recommendations for progression, drawing on your records and other resources; and
- work in partnership with the practice assessor to evaluate and recommend the student for progression for each part of the programme.

(NMC, 2018c, p11)

Your academic assessor will be familiar with your programme of study and is allocated by your university. Their role is to check that your practice assessor is an appropriately prepared registered nurse, that they acknowledged any feedback from your practice supervisor, and have conducted a fair, objective assessment of your performance. They will also check that you have been provided with the opportunity to receive feedback for further development during your placement.

These new roles have been introduced by the NMC in response to 'failing to fail' concerns.

---

### Research summary: Failing to fail

Duffy's (2003) seminal work on failure to fail identified the reluctance on the part of mentors to fail a student in practice. Her work was supported by a number of studies that reported an unwillingness of mentors to fail students, particularly when the student's performance was borderline or they felt unsupported in making such an important decision (Lankshear, 1990; Duffy, 2003, 2006; Hunt et al., 2012). Some research reported that students were five times more likely to fail their academic studies than fail practice (Hunt et al., 2012) and some mentors reported they felt intimidated by students' coercive behaviours (Hunt et al., 2014).

---

The introduction of the multiple roles – practice supervisor, practice assessor and academic assessor – aims to ensure a more balanced approach to the way you are supervised and assessed in practice by enabling a collaborative approach between the practice supervisor, practice assessor and academic assessor. The practice supervisor will facilitate your learning, identifying learning opportunities to help you achieve the necessary NMC proficiencies/professional values (NMC, 2018e). They will then feed back on your progress to the practice assessor, who will undertake assessment of your competence. The role of the academic assessor is to ensure that there is evidence that an accurate and fair assessment has been performed. Your university programme guide/course handbook will inform you as to how many parts there are in your programme and who your academic assessor will be for each part.

# Other supporting roles

In addition to these new roles, there are a number of other roles that can provide support to you while on your placement.

## Personal tutor

You will be allocated a personal tutor while you are on the programme. Your programme guide/course handbook will identify the responsibilities of a personal tutor, but they are primarily there to support you pastorally, academically and professionally throughout your programme. Their role will include scrutiny of your Practice Assessment Document (PAD) and guidance, or referral to additional support services, such as academic skills, special education assessment/support, or the mental well-being team if required. If you are aware that you are experiencing problems that might impact on your performance or attendance in placement, you should seek their support. An example of how a personal tutor supporting a student or making referrals to specialist services can help when problems impact on placement can be seen in Amy's case study.

---

### Case study: Amy

I came to realise the importance of a good support network when I faced personal difficulties over the two years of my MSc Adult Nursing course. Initially, I avoided contacting my personal tutor as I felt embarrassed about my situation and could not see how she would be able to help me, but I began to feel increasingly anxious and distressed, so I texted her and briefly explained my situation. We agreed to meet up, and I was so relieved we did, as she referred me to the university well-being team and occupational health services, and I was able to access counselling services. I remained in regular contact with my personal tutor and valued the well-being services, as when things were increasingly difficult, I could drop in for a chat or access

*(Continued)*

---

(Continued)

the counsellor. However, there came a point when my personal life started to impact on my health and performance in practice, and I realised I needed a break. Although at the time it was difficult to rationalise my decision to interrupt my studies (with only two months to go to the end of my programme and halfway through my final placement), I was surprised at the great sense of relief when my personal tutor explained the processes of interruption, and I finally made my decision to interrupt. During my interruption, my personal tutor and I kept in regular contact, and when I felt fit to return I met with my personal tutor, and we discussed when would be a good time and if I needed any additional support services to enable me to feel supported in practice. It is now one year on, and I am back and am coming to the end of my final placement. My personal tutor and the practice staff, including the practice educators, have been amazing. My personal tutor has been in regular contact while on placement, the link lecturer has been to visit me to check I am being supported, and the practice educators have overseen my supervision in placement by offering drop-in services if I am feeling stressed. I am near to the end of my final placement and I am about to be assessed; it is anticipated that I will pass, and I will finally become a registered nurse! My journey has been a challenging one, but it has taught me a great deal about looking after myself and others, as well as accessing support when things are difficult.

You can see above that Amy was able to access support from her personal tutor when she was experiencing difficulty. There are many ways in which one can access support, and sometimes face-to-face is more difficult. Like Amy, you might feel embarrassed, particularly if information is sensitive or you feel emotional. Take a moment to consider Activity 4.2.

## Activity 4.2   Communication

Think of the different ways in which you could make contact with your personal tutor.

How might you pluck up the courage to share private information with them?

How might they respond?

What might be the consequences if you don't ask for support?

*An outline answer to parts of this activity is given at the end of the chapter.*

You can see from Amy's case study that she initially did not know what to say to her personal tutor, or how she might help with her situation, but by seeking support she was able to make informed decisions that influenced her return to placement and her eventual success. In addition to her personal tutor, Amy explained how the link lecturer and practice education team supported her on placement. Let's look at how these roles can help you to be successful in your placement.

# Academic support to practice

Universities usually have a system whereby designated members of the academic team support students and practice staff in placement areas. Each university uses different titles (e.g. link lecturers, liaison lecturers, clinical teachers). They will be informed when you are being allocated to the practice area that they are responsible for and will oversee your placement experience. If you are experiencing any difficulties or have any questions that your practice supervisor, assessor or educator (see below) cannot answer, your link lecturer should be your first point of contact. If you cannot get hold of them, your personal tutor or academic assessor should be your next point of contact. Leyla's case study is an example of where a student used the support of both the link lecturer and personal tutor to help them cope with difficulties in placement.

---

## Case study: Leyla

Leyla has experienced anxiety throughout the programme and has accessed the well-being team at regular intervals. She is experiencing personal and financial difficulty and has attempted her final placement twice, but due to stress has gone off sick and interrupted from the programme on one occasion. Leyla is halfway through her final placement when the practice assessor contacts the link lecturer to say that Leyla is not performing to the required level. The link lecturer visits both the student and practice assessor in the placement area and facilitates a discussion. Leyla feels overwhelmed by the feedback and goes off sick. The link lecturer informs Leyla's personal tutor, who makes contact with Leyla, and they discuss how her mental health is being affected by the feedback. Leyla informs her personal tutor that she wants to withdraw from the programme. Leyla's personal tutor rings her up and asks her to agree to a referral to occupational health for assessment. Occupational health confirms Leyla is not fit for practice and refers her for cognitive behavioural therapy. Leyla finds this really helpful, and when occupational health confirms Leyla is fit to return, the personal tutor liaises with the practice learning team at the university, who identify an appropriate new placement area. The university finance services were able to offer Leyla some funds to help her pay her rent and she is now doing really well in placement. The link lecturer for this area is supporting both Leyla and her new practice assessor, and Leyla is expected to pass her final placement. Leyla's personal tutor has been in regular contact via email and is pleased with Leyla's progress.

---

You can see from Leyla's case study that some students really struggle in placement. Their mental health can be impacted by a number of things, and the link lecturer and personal tutor are key to the student's success, as are the practice educators based in practice who work closely with the academic staff from the university and practice assessors and supervisors. We have touched on the practice educator several times; now let's explore how they will support you in placement.

## Practice educators

This is an experienced member of the practice team who oversees and supports the practice supervisors and assessors across a group of placements within the organisation in which they are employed. They will be able to resolve many issues that your practice supervisor and assessor cannot, or you can contact them if you feel you need more support. They work closely with the staff from university and are often responsible for coordinating student placements.

## Organisation education leads

Each organisation has an education lead; this is a senior member of the education team/organisation who is responsible for the overall coordination and management of practice learning for both students and qualified/unqualified staff within the organisation. They have a key role in managing the student experience and working in collaboration with the university and other organisations in relation to education, recruitment, retention and training.

## Student support services

As a student, there might be times when you need some additional support. For example, you may have specific learning needs, such as dyslexia, or suffer with anxiety, and therefore need support in preparing for your placement or additional support while you are out on placement. If you require reasonable adjustments, you should ensure that the placement team or the lead for practice at the university are aware so they can consider if your reasonable adjustments can be met on your planned placement. It is, however, your responsibility to communicate your reasonable adjustments with your practice supervisor and assessor; while you do not have to share confidential information with the practice staff, you are encouraged to do so to ensure you get the full range of support you need. Your university will have a range of support services that you might have accessed when you started the programme or you can be referred to if there is a need. Your personal tutor/academic linking to practice can advise you or you can access the services directly. We will explore this area further in Chapter 8, but let's consider how you might respond to a student who needs support as described in the case study below.

This situation may be quite daunting for you, so consider how you would respond by completing Activity 4.3.

---

### Case study: Emily

Emily is a first-year student on her first placement. This is the first time she has been away from home and she is finding it all overwhelming. She confides in you as a third-year student that she previously suffered from an eating disorder and self-harm, and although she has been coping she is now feeling increasingly down and is not sleeping.

---

### Activity 4.3   Communication

1.  What should you advise Emily?
2.  What do you think you can do to support Emily?

*An outline answer to this activity is given at the end of the chapter.*

---

As you progress through your course, you will find that junior students will look to you more often for guidance and support. Your peers are another form of support available to you.

## Peer support

Fellow students will have a better insight and understanding into how you feel, and as they are not your supervisor or assessor, you will feel more able to share things with them than with your supervisor or assessor, who you may believe will judge you more negatively. Supporting other students is good practice for when you take on the role of practice supervisor after you qualify.

# Getting the best support in placement

Sometimes it is difficult to see the relevance of the placement to your learning needs. There are a range of people who might be able to help you see the learning opportunities available. These might include other students, your practice supervisor/assessor, or the practice educator for that area. The following scenario has been designed to help you think about how you might deal with certain situations in placement.

## Scenario: When your placement doesn't start well

You have been looking forward to commencing your placement, and you have explored the types of patients/service users that are cared for in this area. However, when you arrive, the staff advise they are not expecting you and they do not have a practice assessor to support you.

Unfortunately, the scenario above is not uncommon. Occasionally, there is a breakdown in communication between your university and the placement provider. Most problems can be easily resolved, so if you find your practice area is not expecting you, then contact your university placements team, the practice educator or your link lecturer/academic assessor. Try not to get anxious or let this experience influence the remainder of your placement or future placements. There will also be times when you feel under-confident or even scared, and you may possibly not feel supported sufficiently by your practice supervisor or assessor. What is essential is to seek help from someone as soon as possible so that support can be put in place. Activity 4.4 asks you to reflect on your experience of support in practice.

## Activity 4.4 Reflection

If you have already had placements, reflect on your interactions so far with your practice supervisors and assessors:

- What went well and what did not go well?
- What skills and attributes have you found make a good practice supervisor?
- Which of these do you believe you possess?
- Which ones do you need to develop?

*As this activity is based on your own experiences, there is no outline answer at the end of the chapter.*

When reflecting on your previous placements, you might want to consider some of the things you did well, such as planning ahead and demonstrating motivation to learn new things. However, be honest with yourself. Could you have read up more on the types of conditions you saw or the services available for these patients/service users? You may have identified a practice supervisor or assessor that inspired you and wish to see how you could develop those skills in yourself. You might also have experienced a situation that made you recognise how you might need to develop the skills to raise any concerns you might witness. Reflection is an important element of learning. It is important that you reflect on your placement experience to help identify your achievements and the areas for development as practice equates to 50 per cent of your programme, so it is as important as your academic marks.

# Assessment of your practice

Your programme will be designed so your knowledge, skills and attitudes are assessed in practice. You will have a competency/proficiency document, usually referred to as a Practice Assessment Document (PAD), and your university will guide you on how you will be assessed in each placement. As discussed earlier, your practice assessor will complete your assessment, supported by the practice supervisor(s), with the whole process overseen by the academic assessor. This does not mean that the academic assessor will necessarily visit you in practice, but if problems arise they may contact/visit you or ask the link lecturer for your area to visit you. If you feel you need support in identifying how to achieve the relevant elements of assessment, you should discuss with your practice supervisor or assessor in the first instance. It is your practice assessor's responsibility to provide you with feedback on your performance. Sometimes feedback can be difficult to receive, so if you are finding this difficult you can discuss this with the practice educator at your placement or your link lecturer/academic assessor. If you feel you have not been treated fairly and an accurate assessment is not being performed, you should contact your link lecturer or academic assessor as soon as possible, as involving them early in the assessment process can prevent problems escalating. We will discuss this in more detail in Chapter 6.

This chapter finishes with a student's message to you.

## Case study: Rochelle

Rochelle is a first-year student. She had been a healthcare assistant for more than ten years; however, when it came to her first placement on the programme, she felt extremely nervous as she had never looked after children before and had been allocated to a children's surgical ward in a very busy London trust. Rochelle reports that she experienced a range of emotions; she was afraid of getting lost, as she had never been to this hospital before, but also frightened of meeting so many new people, and felt a desire to run back to what was familiar. In addition to the fear, Rochelle also felt an element of excitement; she was looking forward to being part of a new team and caring for people's babies and children, helping them on their journey to recovery.

*(Continued)*

(Continued)

Rochelle realised that all her worries and fears were soon to vanish once she had met the qualified staff who were to support her in her placement. They were very kind and understanding, and also helped her to develop her skills, encouraging her to express her fear so they could support her through this stressful period. Rochelle soon recognised that there was a range of people there to help her settle into her placement, not only the nurse who was allocated to her to assess her skills and competence, but also other qualified and unqualified healthcare professionals. She also found it comforting to meet other students on placement as they could offer advice and reassure her that her feelings were normal. All these people contributed to supporting Rochelle on placement, and she shares her story with you to reassure you that it will be OK.

Rochelle's case study shows the importance of letting someone know when you are worried or have problems on placement. There are a multitude of staff as well as other students who can advise and support you.

## Chapter summary

It is hoped that this chapter has provided you with a greater understanding as to how the NMC standards underpin the new roles in supporting you in practice. It is anticipated that the registered practitioners in the roles of practice supervisor and assessor will assist you in putting the theory you have learnt in university, in your own personal study and through discussion into practice, which will help you to achieve the knowledge, skills and attitudes to be a competent registered nurse by the end of your programme.

You will have seen from the case studies and through your participation in the activities that there are a range of people who are keen to help you through any difficult times, and many students have experienced challenges and continued to succeed on the programme. Therefore, the message is: do not suffer in silence, but always seek support, as nursing can be challenging but immensely rewarding.

## Activities: brief outline answers

### Activity 4.1   Critical thinking (p64)

There are a number of people who might support you in your placement. Some of these might not be nurses or other students, but other registered practitioners. These might include doctors, physiotherapists, social workers, speech and language therapists, psychologists, physician assistants and other registered nurses. A teacher is not a registered health and social care practitioner; therefore, they cannot be your practice supervisor, but they can contribute to your learning under the supervision of a practice supervisor or assessor.

## Activity 4.2 Communication (p68)

There are a variety of ways to communicate with your personal tutor, and you should agree the ground rules/parameters when you first meet with them. Examples are text/SMS, WhatsApp, email, mobile phone/landline, or a university-specific closed social media group/chat room. Note that it is not appropriate for you to become 'friends' with your personal tutor/practice staff on non-university social media as this might compromise your professional relationship.

Your personal tutor will be able to advise or guide you to specialist support at the university. It is important to remember that situations are likely to feel better if you share and access support, and ignoring them is not an effective strategy, and is likely to make you feel even more anxious.

## Activity 4.3 Communication (p71)

1.  You could suggest she talks to her personal tutor (or any member of staff she feels is approachable) about her past history and how she is feeling now, or she could visit the student support services at the university. Most universities will have a well-being centre and/or mental health advisors, and anything she shares with them will be totally confidential.

2.  Give Emily time to talk about how she is feeling; listening rather than trying to find answers will be very helpful to her. If you have serious concerns about her well-being, you may need to share your concerns with a member of the teaching team; ideally, get her permission to talk with someone.

## Further reading

**Lidster, J. and Wakefield, S.** (2019) *Student Practice Supervision and Assessment.* London: SAGE.

Aimed at staff in practice, this is a good overview of the new roles and approach to supervision and assessment in practice.

## Useful websites

Pan London Practice Learning Group

**https://plplg.uk**

There is a wealth of resources available on this website, which you can use to familiarise yourself and others about the new roles discussed in this chapter.

NMC: Supporting Information on Standards for Student Supervision and Assessment

**www.nmc.org.uk/supporting-information-on-standards-for-student-supervision-and-assessment/**

The NMC has a web page with a series of guides on the new roles described in this chapter. The guide on student empowerment is particularly good.

Royal College of Nursing: Advice Guides for Students

**www.rcn.org.uk/get-help/rcn-advice/student-nurses**

A series of short guides for student nurses on a range of topics, including placements, accountability and raising concerns.

# Chapter 5

# How to get the most out of your placement

Karen Elcock

## NMC Standards of Proficiency for Registered Nurses

This chapter will address the following platforms and proficiencies:

**Platform 1: Being an accountable professional**

Registered nurses act in the best interests of people, putting them first and providing nursing care that is person-centred, safe and compassionate. They act professionally at all times and use their knowledge and experience to make evidence-based decisions about care. They communicate effectively, are role models for others, and are accountable for their actions. Registered nurses continually reflect on their practice and keep abreast of new and emerging developments in nursing, health and care.

At the point of registration, the registered nurse will be able to:

1.8   demonstrate the knowledge, skills and ability to think critically when applying evidence and drawing on experience to make evidence informed decisions in all situations.

1.10 demonstrate resilience and emotional intelligence and be capable of explaining the rationale that influences their judgements and decisions in routine, complex and challenging situations.

1.17 take responsibility for continuous self-reflection, seeking and responding to support and feedback to develop their professional knowledge and skills.

1.18 demonstrate the knowledge and confidence to contribute effectively and proactively in an interdisciplinary team.

**Platform 6: Improving safety and quality of care**

Registered nurses make a key contribution to the continuous monitoring and quality improvement of care and treatment in order to enhance health outcomes and people's experience of nursing and related care. They assess risks to safety or experience and take appropriate action to manage those, putting the best interests, needs and preferences of people first.

At the point of registration, the registered nurse will be able to:

6.11 acknowledge the need to accept and manage uncertainty, and demonstrate an understanding of strategies that develop resilience in self and others.
6.12 understand the role of registered nurses and other health and care professionals at different levels of experience and seniority when managing and prioritising actions and care in the event of a major incident.

## Chapter aims

After reading this chapter, you will be able to:

- develop strategies that enable you to join the community of practice;
- consider the role that patients/service users, carers and members of the multi-disciplinary team can play in enhancing your learning;
- identify outreach opportunities that add value to your learning;
- explore potential problems that may arise and how to manage them; and
- appreciate the importance of evaluating your learning experience.

# Introduction

## Case study: The proactive student

Many years ago, I was visiting a cardiac ward I linked with and met up with a group of students who were nearing the end of their placement. I asked them how their placement had been going. Three moaned that they hadn't done very much and seemed to spend most of their time washing patients and doing observations and had felt like healthcare assistants. The fourth student, Jenna, smiled, shook her head and said that she had had an amazing experience. She had been involved in caring for acutely ill patients, completed several admissions, accompanied patients to different departments and stayed with them while they were having investigations. The other students looked amazed and asked how she had managed to do so much. Jenna simply said

*(Continued)*

(Continued)

she had asked. She would listen carefully to handover at the start of the shift to see what was going on and would then ask to be involved in a new admission or to take a patient for their angiogram. She would listen out during the day, and if she heard something needed doing or happening elsewhere on the ward she would volunteer to help, or if it was something she could not do herself she would ask if she could go and watch the nurse/doctor doing it.

This chapter has started with the above real-life story as it encapsulates so well the important part you play in your own learning. Jenna and the other students had experienced completely different learning experiences on the same ward, and this was primarily because Jenna actively looked out for learning opportunities and asked to be involved. While on placement, you will work alongside a range of people who will help plan and supervise your learning, but they are also busy looking after the patients/service users in their care. There is therefore an expectation from them that you will take some responsibility for your own learning and be proactive in seeking out further learning opportunities to enhance your placement experience. This chapter will look at the importance of identifying what you need to learn and how you can maximise the learning on each placement by exploring the different learning opportunities available to you. Sometimes a placement does not always go to plan, so common problems will be explored, and we will look at some of the strategies you can use to manage them.

# First impressions

We have touched on this in Chapter 2, but it is important to understand that a poor impression on the first day will take some time to set right, so making sure you turn up on time and are appropriately dressed, with your Practice Assessment Document and any other equipment/information the placement may expect you to bring, will always make a positive impression. Staff will expect you to be nervous, but try to smile and introduce yourself, being clear who you are and what year of the programme you are in. If it is your very first placement, then it is important that you tell them that.

If you have undertaken preparation for your placement, as we discussed in Chapter 2, you will have an idea of the types of learning opportunities your placement will offer, which will allow you to plan ahead before you meet with your practice supervisor and assessor to discuss your learning objectives for the placement. Having considered what it is that you want to focus on learning before you arrive on your placement will impress your practice supervisor/assessor and allow for a far more focused initial interview than simply handing your Practice Assessment Document over and expecting them to read through it all and identify everything you need to learn. It demonstrates interest and a willingness to learn, and this, along with active participation, is essential in order to join the community of nursing practice. While you are supernumerary, the staff in practice are not, so time is precious, and preparation from you before you start can pay dividends in showing you are interested, as well as ensuring that your time with them is used to your best advantage.

We discussed the NMC's definition of 'supernumerary' in Chapter 1. The definition makes clear that your role in practice is to 'learn to provide safe and effective care, not merely to observe' (NMC, 2018d, p18). Therefore, engaging in caregiving is essential. It not only allows you to develop and hone the skills you will need as a registered nurse, but also enables you to participate as a member of the team. This in turn will develop your sense of 'belongingness', which is strongly linked with student satisfaction on placement (Borrott et al., 2016). Initially, you may feel like an outsider as the staff will speak in what often sounds like a foreign language, and while they are familiar with the local rules and routines of a working day, you may have little idea as to what to expect unless you have worked in a similar environment before. While any shift has a series of activities that have to take place in an expected order, healthcare is invariably messy and unpredictable. Events can happen that are not planned for and require an ability to be flexible and responsive to meet the needs of patients and those around you. What this means is that while you can plan to undertake certain learning activities during the course of a shift, you should always be prepared to reconsider these if unplanned events take place. Conversely, learning to adapt to unpredicted or rapidly changing events as they arise (e.g. a cardiac arrest or the need to divert to see a service user in crisis) is a useful skill to develop as a nurse.

# Identifying your learning objectives

For your first placement, it is not unusual to feel that you need to know and learn everything as quickly as possible. The reality is that you can never learn everything there is about nursing, even by the end of your course. Learning in nursing is a lifelong experience, and each class at university and every placement you attend will contribute to your store of knowledge. Pre-registration nursing programmes cover a wide range of subjects and their aim is to ensure that you meet the *Standards of Proficiency for Registered Nurses* set by the NMC (2018e) by the end of the programme. It is unlikely that any programme will fully prepare you for the speciality that you gain your first post in, hence the need for **preceptorship** when you qualify to help you with that transition and support your further learning (Whitehead, 2013).

So, when planning for your placement, there are two important considerations: deciding what you *need* to learn and what you *want* to learn. The first will be dictated by your Practice Assessment Document, which will have a number of learning outcomes/proficiencies/skills that you need to complete in order to pass practice. Your practice supervisor may also identify some additional skills specific to the placement you are on. Added to this may be areas for development identified from your previous placement or learning outcomes you failed on a previous placement that must be passed on this next one. Then there are additional skills or learning opportunities you want to engage with because you have a particular interest in developing expertise in them. However, while the latter can enhance your experience, they should not take priority over the essential ones in your Practice Assessment Document that have to be achieved in order for you to progress. We will look at the assessment process in more detail in the Chapter 6, but try Activity 5.1 to get you started in thinking about what you need to learn.

## Activity 5.1   Critical thinking

Read through your Practice Assessment Document and identify:

- what you have already learnt through classes in skills and simulation, and prioritise those that you feel you need to practise further;
- topics that have been covered in class as theory that will help you to achieve specific proficiencies in practice;
- any areas in your assessment document you don't understand; and
- if you have already completed one or more placements, list any areas you need to improve on based on the feedback you received.

*As this activity is based on your own experience and knowledge, there is no outline answer at the end of the chapter.*

For the last two points, you may need some help in exploring these before you go out to practice. Point 3 may be covered as part of preparation for practice, but you may not wish to discuss the feedback you have had in front of others, so arrange to meet with your personal tutor to discuss the feedback you have received, and if anything is still unclear in your Practice Assessment Document discuss that as well. You should now have a list of skills, activities and areas you want/need to focus on for your placement that you can use as a starting point at your initial interview, and this is sure to impress your practice supervisor.

# Who can you learn from?

You will spend a lot of your time working alongside qualified nurses, but there are many other people you can learn from while on placement. In fact, on some placements, you may have one or more practice supervisors who are not nurses. This is supported by the NMC, who define a practice supervisor as any registered healthcare professional (NMC, 2018c). Working with other health professionals will help you to gain a wider experience of how different professionals work together. Every practice setting will provide opportunities to learn with and from other people, the variety depending on the speciality and field of practice. For example, learning disability students may be placed in a special school and work alongside teachers, speech and language therapists, and physiotherapists. Activity 5.2 helps you to identify the variety of people you may work with.

## Activity 5.2   Team working

List all of the people other than nurses that are involved in the care of patients, service users and children that you are aware of or who you have had an opportunity to meet/work alongside when on placement.

*An outline answer to this activity is given at the end of the chapter.*

Did you include patients and service users or healthcare assistants in your list? These two groups play a significant role in student learning, and yet are not always considered as a learning resource by students. Let's look at how they can contribute to your learning in more detail.

# Patients and service users

Patients and service users are an important source of learning not just because by participating in their care you can practise your clinical skills or nursing interventions, but because they can also provide you with a wealth of information about their personal experiences. Many are experts in their condition, and they can offer you insights into their journey through the healthcare system and the impact of their health condition on their day-to-day life. As you build a trusting relationship with them, you can explore how they have coped (or not) with the challenges they have faced, and will find this enables you to develop a greater insight and understanding of their experiences and use that knowledge to help you when caring for other patients or service users with similar diagnoses or in similar situations. You will find that most patients and service users will be happy to talk with you and share their experiences. This is described well by a patient who said:

*I feel very isolated being in a side room and I am quite a social person so you know her [a nurse] coming in here to talk to me about it and be with me for a while just made me feel so much better.*

(Bramley and Matiti, 2014, p2796)

One of the benefits of being a student is the amount of time you can spend listening to and empathising with the people you care for. It can, however, be quite nerve-wracking to approach someone you don't know for the first time and start up a conversation with them, but there are a number of approaches you can use.

An easy way is simply to talk to them while giving care (e.g. when helping them with their hygiene needs, taking observations, helping them with their food, changing a dressing, or by participating in a game or activity with them). Alternatively, if you find yourself with some 'free' time, then approach one of your patients/service users, tell them you are a student, and ask them if they would be happy to talk to you about why they are in hospital/at the clinic and what their experiences have been like. If you're not sure who to approach, ask one of the staff on your placement who they think would be happy to talk to you or who they think might have a particularly interesting experience to share with you. The following case study describes Dev's experience talking with a service user in the community. Read through it, noting his approach to communicating with the service user, and then complete Activity 5.3.

## Case study: Dev

Dev is on a community placement and has been practising his aseptic technique by doing a number of dressings for people who have leg ulcers. He has met Mary before. She is a middle-aged lady with a learning disability who has had her leg ulcer for several months and finds the dressing changes very painful. Dev asks his practice supervisor if he can sit and talk with Mary while she does the dressing. He asks Mary if she is happy to talk to him about her leg while it is being dressed and she says she'd love to tell him all about it. Dev pulls up a chair and sits squarely near her, leaning forward and using eye contact to show his interest in her. By the time his practice assessor has finished the dressing, Dev has found out that Mary finds her leg ulcer distressing, it is so painful that she rarely goes for walks to the park any more with her sister, and she says her ulcer smells awful. Mary looks tearful as she says she has heard people saying she smells when she goes to the day centre; as a consequence, she says she doesn't want to go there any more. Mary's sister, who is sitting with them, says this would mean she would never get time to herself. She also complains about the extra washing she has to do because Mary's leg ulcer leaks through the dressing. When Dev got home, he reflected on Mary and her sister and the impact that Mary's leg ulcer had on them both. He had never considered how much it could adversely affect a person's life and the lives of people around them.

## Activity 5.3   Communication

What skills did Dev use to encourage Mary to talk, which helped her to feel secure enough to open up and share her feelings with him?

*An outline answer to this activity is given at the end of the chapter.*

Dev's approach with Mary is a good example of effective communication skills. He could have started with some small talk first, asking Mary how she was feeling or commenting on the weather or a picture in the room. If you have access to a person's notes, there may be information on their hobbies or other details you can ask them about that will help break the ice.

From this experience, Dev gained a first-hand understanding of the impact that a chronic leg ulcer had on both Mary and her sister. Mary suffered from pain, exudate, odour and mobility problems, leading to social isolation. Following on from this, Dev should now read about the pathophysiology of venous leg ulcers to understand how they are caused, and he could also explore the research on the psychosocial impact of leg ulcers. For example, the problems identified by Mary and her sister have all been identified in a systematic review by Green et al. (2014) as common factors that impact on the quality of a person's life. This study recommends that the problems a patient has need to be discussed at each visit/consultation if they are ever to be addressed effectively. Having read this research, Dev will now ensure he discusses the wider problems the people he meets who have a leg ulcer may be having, rather than just focusing on the ulcer itself. He also knows now that it must include liaising with the multidisciplinary team to find solutions that can improve their quality of life. The importance of not taking things at face value also applies to the people you work with; healthcare assistants are a particular case.

## Healthcare assistants

Student evaluations of their placements sometimes reveal that they feel they spend too much time with healthcare assistants (HCAs). This view is supported in a number of studies exploring the experience of students and HCAs in practice (e.g. Hasson et al., 2013; Gillespie and Rivers, 2017). Some students also report that they feel they are involved in delivering what they perceive as too much basic care on some placement. It is this that can add to their perception that they are treated like an HCA rather than a student. This view, however, shows a lack of understanding of the importance of what are not basic skills, but fundamental nursing skills that are essential to good patient care. As an example, Table 5.1 lists some of the information you can gain about a person during a bed bath or helping them with their hygiene needs.

| What you can observe | What it may indicate |
|---|---|
| Visual inspection – emaciated | Poor nutritional status |
| Skin temperature | High – potential infection |
| | Low – poor circulation |
| Breathing pattern | Laboured breathing – respiratory infection, hypoxic |
| Lack of skin turgor/dry skin and/or dry oral mucosa | Can indicate dehydration |
| Loss of muscle mass and/or red heels/sacrum/elbows | Low level of activity |
| | At risk of pressure ulcers |
| Evidence of rashes | Allergies, including an allergic response to antibiotics |
| | Skin conditions such as psoriasis, eczema |
| | Rashes can also be signs of more serious conditions such as shingles or sepsis |
| Difficulty in moving or guarding of parts of the body | May indicate pain and needs investigating to determine the cause |
| Mental status | Signs of anxiety, depression, dementia |
| | A confusional state can be a sign of infection, particularly in the elderly |

*Table 5.1*   Learning from fundamental skills

Nurses use and apply their knowledge of normal physiology, pathophysiology and the behavioural sciences when delivering care. Using this knowledge, they can learn a lot about a person's physical and mental health status and make initial diagnoses, all while delivering these fundamental skills. It is also important to note that the Mid Staffordshire hospital scandal (Francis, 2013), which raised concerns regarding failures in fundamental care, highlighted that fundamental care was the responsibility of all staff.

Historically, the HCA role was implemented to replace the contribution that student nurses gave in practice when nurse education moved into universities in the 1990s and students became supernumerary. Over time, HCAs have become the backbone of the NHS, delivering the majority of direct care. The research study summarised below offers the perspective of HCAs on their role when working with and supporting student nurses. The research has some interesting findings, which you may or may not agree with. Once you have read it, complete Activity 5.4.

## Research summary: The role of healthcare assistants in supporting student learning in practice

The research study by Hasson et al. (2013) was undertaken in Northern Ireland and explored the role of the HCA in supporting student nurse learning in clinical practice. It identified how HCAs played a major role in both supporting and teaching student nurses because they often worked alongside students more than the registered nurses who were the named mentors/supervisors/assessors of students. The 'teaching' that HCAs were involved in focused on direct care but in some areas could also include technical and specialist tasks. While many students might be allocated to an HCA, some students would make a point of choosing to work alongside them, seeing it as an opportunity to be involved in direct care.

## Activity 5.4   Critical thinking

What are your views regarding HCAs or other unqualified staff supporting and teaching students? If you have already had a placement, what was your own experience?

*As this activity is based on your own views, there is no outline answer at the end of the chapter.*

Undoubtedly, your view on the value of working with HCAs will depend on a number of factors: whether you have been an HCA yourself before, your experience of working with them as a student so far, what stage of the programme you are on, and the experience and skill sets of the HCAs you have had contact with. In the *Shape of Caring* review led by Lord Willis, HCAs were found to deliver more than 60 per cent of hands-on care (HEE, 2015). It will therefore not be surprising for you to often work alongside an HCA, who will not only involve you in a range of direct care activities that you will want to learn about and practise, but in doing so you will also be provided with lots of opportunities to talk with patients and service users. These opportunities are essential in developing your skills and confidence as a nurse. You may also be surprised to find that many HCAs have extended their skill set and taken on technical tasks that were once only undertaken by doctors and nurses, such as venepuncture, phlebotomy, 12-lead ECGs, taking observations, monitoring blood glucose and dressing some wounds, and they may even run clinics. Therefore, by working alongside them, they can offer additional and sometimes unexpected learning opportunities for you.

## Other health and social care professionals

It is an NMC expectation that nursing students learn with and from other health and social care professionals (HSCPs). This allows you to gain a more holistic understanding of how healthcare is delivered and the roles of other people in the care and treatment of the people you will be caring for. An ageing population and an increasing number of people with long-term conditions or co-morbidities means that many people using the health service will be cared for by more than one HSCP. By spending time with them, you can gain an understanding of their roles and how the effectiveness of each is so dependent on how well we all work together and communicate to each other. As the person who often spends the most time with patients or service users, in both hospital and community settings, the nurse is central to effective interprofessional collaboration and multi-agency working, and the NMC have clearly articulated the importance of your role in working with and across professional groups within their latest standards of proficiency (NMC, 2018e). The best way of learning about the roles of other HCSPs is to spend time with them, and this can be achieved through attending multidisciplinary team meetings or undertaking 'spoke', outreach or insight placements with different HSCPs who are involved in the care of the people on your placement. The next section describes these short placement experiences and how they can be arranged.

# Outreach, insight or hub-and-spoke placements

Many universities will offer hub-and-spoke placements or encourage you to arrange and undertake outreach or insight placements yourself. These can provide you with opportunities to explore the patient/service user journey and develop a greater understanding of their experience of the healthcare system. They also offer opportunities, as touched on above, to meet with and develop an understanding of the role that different health and social care practitioners and other services play in the patient/service user journey.

A hub relates to your base/main placement from which you then go out on a series of shorter placements, called spokes. You may do one or more hub placements in a year or you may have one hub placement stretched across a whole academic year, with a series of different spokes each time you return to it from university. These types of placements are usually formalised by the university in conjunction with the placement in advance, with the spokes lasting from a week to several weeks, depending on the length of the whole placement (McClimens and Brewster, 2017).

Outreach or insight placements, on the other hand, tend to be more ad hoc and can be influenced by your own interests and the type of placement you are on. They can last a few hours to a couple of days and should always be linked to the speciality of the placement (e.g. following a patient to theatres while on a surgical placement, spending time with the **enuresis nurse specialist** while on a children's community placement, spending time with an art therapist on a mental health or learning disability placement). Your practice supervisor/assessor may suggest relevant outreach activities that you can undertake on your placement. However, you can also play a part in identifying appropriate learning opportunities by undertaking some research in advance about your placement and identifying the potential opportunities that may be available. What is important is that any outreach placement/activity must have relevance to the placement you are on. For example, spending a day in the maternity unit when your main placement is in an elderly care ward is not relevant, but it may be relevant if you are on a gynaecology ward. Steps you can take to identify outreach activities are:

- Talk to the people in your care about their healthcare journey to identify who has been involved in their care. This will help you to identify other health and social care professionals you could spend time with.
- Ask the team on your placement what specialist nurses and other healthcare professionals are involved in the care of their client group.
- Find out what other departments or organisations people on your placement may be sent/referred to for investigations, treatment or therapies.

Once you have completed the above, compile a list of people and departments who are involved in the care of your client group. Use this as a focus for discussion with your practice supervisor to decide who it may be appropriate to spend a half-day/day with and then agree a timetable of outreach activities, ensuring that the majority of your time is still on your main placement and allows sufficient time to meet with your practice assessor at key points during your placement. If you spend too much time away from your main placement, then you may run into difficulties in getting your Practice Assessment Document completed. Table 5.2 provides some examples of spokes that may be available to you on different types of placement.

| Hub or main placement | Spokes, outreach, insight |
| --- | --- |
| In-hospital placements (adult and child) | Pre-operative assessment clinic |
| | Theatres – time with anaesthetist, surgeon, operating department practitioners, theatre/recovery nurses |
| | Outpatients departments |
| | Radiography – X-ray, CT scans, MRIs, angiography |
| | Clinical nurse specialists (e.g. stoma, breast care, infection control, diabetes) |
| | Pain clinics |
| | Midwifery unit |
| Community placements | Practice nurse |
| | Health visitors |
| | Community midwives |
| | Clinical nurse specialists |
| | Chiropodist |
| | GP |
| | Day centres, care homes, nursing homes |
| Children's nursing | **Child and adolescent mental health services (CAMHS)** |
| | Mental health school link worker |
| | Neonatal outreach nurse |
| | Nurseries |
| Mental health | Mental health school link worker |
| | Mental health charities/voluntary groups |
| | Clinical psychologist |

*(Continued)*

*Table 5.2*   (Continued)

| Hub or main placement | Spokes, outreach, insight |
|---|---|
| Learning disability | Housing providers<br><br>Charities/voluntary groups that support people with a learning disability and their families |
| All fields | Safeguarding teams<br>Clinical risk teams<br>Hospital discharge team<br>Social work team<br>Research nurses<br>Resuscitation team<br>Chaplaincy<br>Healthcare professionals (e.g. physiotherapist, occupational therapist, dietician, pharmacists, paramedics) |

*Table 5.2*   Spoke or outreach placements and activities

Insight placements can be spokes or outreach placements but are often used to describe time with patients/service users from a different field of practice. For example, an adult student on a community placement with a district nurse spends some time with a health visitor visiting families and children, and a child field student on a community placement could spend time with the diabetes specialist nurse visiting adults in order to gain an insight into the longer-term impact of diabetes when it is not well controlled, which can inform their education of children who are diagnosed with the disease.

# Self-initiated learning

There are many activities you can organise yourself to help with your learning. These can be integrated into your day or undertaken when there is some 'quiet' time. For example, you will need to develop your knowledge of pharmacology and an understanding of the medications prescribed for the people you will be caring for. Your university cannot teach you about every drug, just the common ones. So, on each placement, select three or four patients/service users, review their notes and drug chart (if they have one) or discuss the medications they are on if in the community, and compile a medication profile as follows:

- Patient/service user diagnosis (don't record names).
- Look on the **National Institute for Health and Care Excellence (NICE)** website (**www.nice.org.uk**) to see if there are any guidelines on recommended medications for the relevant diagnosis.
- List the medications prescribed. How do these match the NICE guidelines, if they exist?

- Why is each medication prescribed? Relate to diagnosis above and NICE guidelines.
- What are the common side effects/contraindications for each?
- Is the patient/service user having any problems with any of their medications? Talk to them about their experiences of taking different drugs.
- e any specific observations you need to take to monitor the effect of the on?

Y able to get a copy of the **British National Formulary (BNF)** on placement or use their website (**https://bnf.nice.org.uk**) to help you with the above.

This approach, linked to real people, is a far better way of learning about medications than trying to learn a long list of them. You will find you remember them if you can link them in your memory to someone you have cared for.

Other activities you can initiate on your own that will help you link practice to theory, and vice versa, which can also benefit staff and students in your placement, as well as patients, carers or service users, are:

- making a list of common conditions, abbreviations and treatments in your placement, and providing short definitions and explanations of each that can then be used for future students;
- developing information leaflets/posters suitable for your client group if none already exist;
- researching an unusual condition and providing a summary or links to resources for staff/students;
- volunteering to assist with patient surveys or clinical audits; and
- writing reflections on your practice experiences (see Chapter 10).

All of the above will demonstrate willingness to learn and are likely to enhance your overall experience. However, sometimes things don't always go to plan. In the next section, we look at common problems that can arise on placement, starting with a case study of a student who had problems, followed by Activity 5.5, which asks you how you would respond if you had problems.

# When problems arise

## Case study: Sara

Sara is struggling with managing her shifts on her placement. Her mother has had to go away to look after Sara's grandmother, who is ill, so Sara is expected to look after her younger brothers and sisters. This means taking them to school each day

*(Continued)*

(Continued)

and collecting them at the end of the day. Sara is embarrassed to discuss her personal life with her practice supervisor, but she has already been picked up on her poor timekeeping and been warned she needs to improve in this area if she is to pass her practice assessment.

## Activity 5.5   Communication

If you were having difficulties in practice, are there any situations that you would find it difficult to discuss with your practice supervisor/assessor? If so, who else might you talk with to get help?

*An outline answer to this activity is given at the end of the chapter.*

A common reason for students not doing well in practice is their failure to discuss external factors that are impacting on their ability to fully engage. These may be family commitments such as the care of other dependents or childcare but can also include financial problems making travel to work difficult, health reasons, or an undisclosed disability. There are a number of options open to Sara, but first and foremost is the need for her to talk to someone.

Ideally she should talk to her practice supervisor and assessor so they understand why her timekeeping/attendance is poor. She doesn't need to go into detail if she finds it difficult, but they do need to know that there is a personal reason impacting on her and what she is going to do in response (e.g. talking to someone at the university). This will reassure them that she acknowledges there is a problem and is trying to manage the situation appropriately. If she feels she is unable to discuss her problems at all with the staff in her placement, then she needs to contact someone at her university as a matter of urgency before the situation escalates.

The link lecturer for the placement and her academic assessor, as well as her personal tutor or the lead for practice at the university, are all appropriate people that can advise. This type of problem is not unusual, and the university may well have strategies they can put in place to help her out in the short term. There are also student advisors at the university who may be able to refer her to services that can provide advice or support. These are always confidential.

The key message here is letting people know you have a problem, and as soon as possible. For example, if Sara knew she was going to have problems managing her placement shifts on a short-term basis before she started her placement, there would have been an opportunity for the university to look at options (e.g. a different type of placement with more family-friendly shifts or negotiation of family-friendly shifts on her current placement until her mother is back at home). The details do not need to be disclosed, but a letter can be provided for the placement explaining that there is a need for some adjustments to hours in practice, which will ensure that practice can provide the appropriate support during this time.

Disclosing personal information can be very difficult for some students, and staff in practice and at the university do appreciate that. Sharing some insights into the challenges you are facing can help the staff in your placement to understand why you are having problems. Most staff are very accommodating in trying to help and support students where there are difficulties, but if they don't know you have problems then they will assume you are not interested or don't care, which is not a recipe for success. MacDonald et al. (2016) identified a number of challenges that students face while on placement, including balancing the demands of their personal life with work demands, as Sara found above. Additional challenges that they identified are discussed below.

## Tiredness

It is important that you get sufficient sleep and rest if you are going to be alert on placement. This is essential if you are going to practise safely and effectively and maximise your learning from the opportunities available to you. Twelve-hour shifts are challenging, and if you find them difficult you can ask to undertake more traditional early/late shifts, although you will get less 'free' days each week, so you need to consider the pros and cons. Wherever possible, don't do consecutive 12-hour shifts. If tiredness is the result of the side effects of medication you have been prescribed, then reasonable adjustments can be put in place (we will discuss this in more detail in Chapter 8).

## Time management: studying and completing assignments

While on placement, you will probably have assignments to prepare for and complete, as well as wanting to research areas that you need to explore further in relation to your placement. This will require you to be very organised in planning your time, and a study/work timetable (with time for yourself also planned in) can be really helpful in ensuring you get a balance. If you find that due to other commitments (e.g. work, family) you cannot make the time needed for upcoming assignments, then this needs an urgent discussion with your personal tutor to ensure you meet assessment deadlines and pass your assignments.

## Loneliness and isolation

When you are at university, you have the support of your peers, but on your placement you may find that you are the only one from your cohort there and don't know the other students, or you may even find that you are the only student there. That can make you feel lonely and even isolated. It can also be difficult to meet up with your peers if your shifts don't coincide. Use of social media can be a valuable way of keeping in contact (e.g. a WhatsApp or Facebook group that only includes your peers), but take care in what you discuss, even if it is a private group, as any information can still be shared externally, and, as we discussed in Chapter 1, you could end up in trouble if you post inappropriate comments. Look back at Chapter 1 and reread the advice it provides on the use of social media and how to be safe when using it. Group video chats on apps such as FaceTime can also be helpful in keeping connected with your peers. You may find there are workshops/meetings across a hospital or community setting that are provided to allow students to meet up and discuss their experiences. Check if these are offered and when they are run so you can try to arrange your shifts to coincide with them.

## Conflicting needs

This often arises when you find you are struggling to balance your own learning needs with the needs of the placement to get 'the work' done. For example, there will be occasions when you want to be involved in a specific activity on placement, but the pressure felt by the staff on your placement to get the day-to-day work done may mean you feel conflict between helping out and taking advantage of the learning opportunities that arise, as well as achieving your own personal learning needs. Consider the following case study describing Aran's experience on placement and then complete Activity 5.6.

---

### Case study: Aran

Aran has been on his placement for more than four weeks. He has two weeks left. It is very busy, and so far he has not had any of his proficiencies signed off. He had identified a number of areas he wanted to develop on this placement, particularly around practising the admissions process and undertaking some drug rounds to develop his skills in medication management. Unfortunately, he has not had an opportunity to achieve any of this so far. He has mainly worked alongside HCAs and newly qualified staff, who have been very supportive, but he hasn't felt that he has been stretched in any way. He keeps his ears open at handover at the start of the day and has asked to be involved in scheduled activities, but inevitably staff say they need him to work somewhere else. He was introduced to his practice supervisor and assessor on his first day, but his assessor has been on sick leave since then and his supervisor has been on leave for the last two weeks. He doesn't want to complain as he knows everyone is busy and he wants to 'keep the staff happy', but he is starting to feel quite resentful at losing opportunities to learn.

## Activity 5.6    Critical thinking

What are the issues here?

What actions should Aran have undertaken, and what should he do now?

*An outline answer to this activity is given at the end of the chapter.*

In addition to the answers given at the end of the chapter, it is important to note that Aran could have had more than one practice supervisor, which would have ensured a member of staff was aware of his situation and his learning needs, and could have advocated for him. The manager needed to know early on that there were problems with the lack of support and that he was not making progress with the completion of his Practice Assessment Document. Aran could have approached the manager or asked a member of staff for help or contacted the link lecturer to intervene. Supernumerary status is also potentially an issue here as Aran is feeling that he is missing out on learning opportunities, with the needs of the placement being seen as more important than his learning. While the needs of patients and service users must always be met, if a student finds their own learning needs are being compromised, then they do need to raise concerns. This is always difficult. If it is not resolved with the practice supervisor or assessor, then it may require discussion with the manager and possibly the involvement of the link lecturer.

# Conflict or difficulties with your practice supervisor or assessor

The relationship you have with your practice supervisors and assessors is important and can either positively or negatively impact on your practice experience. It can take time to develop an effective working relationship, and if you are on a short placement then it can be more difficult to build that relationship, particularly if undertaking long days so you are only on duty three or four shifts per week. Table 5.3 lists the attributes that mentors (now practice assessors/supervisors) viewed as important in students.

| Positive attributes | Negative attributes |
|---|---|
| Enthusiastic | Disinterested |
| Interested | Lazy |
| Keen | Overconfident and not willing to listen |
| Students who want to learn | Too focused on their mobile phone |
| | Unmotivated |

*Table 5.3*   Student attributes that mentors viewed positively and negatively

*Source*: Adapted from Rylance et al. (2017, p407)

As you can see, there is a common thread around demonstrating (or not) interest and enthusiasm towards your placement and learning. It is therefore important that you demonstrate interest and a willingness to learn if clinical staff are going to demonstrate a reciprocal interest in helping you to gain the most from your placement. This was discussed at the start of the chapter when we looked at the importance of preparing for your placement, but it is also important to continue to be proactive in your learning. You can do this by identifying learning opportunities, not hanging back when it is particularly busy, and researching and reading around topics relevant to your placement so that you can demonstrate your commitment to learning. However, sometimes the student–practice supervisor/assessor relationship can fail. There can be many reasons for this, so if you are doing your best to show interest and engage, consider what may be happening from your supervisor/assessor's perspective.

Many may feel conflict between supporting you and meeting the needs of patients, and this can make them feel guilty or even angry. This is not personal, but it can make you feel equally guilty when asking for help or guidance, knowing how busy they are. Sometimes there may be cultural misunderstandings. The UK attracts nurses from across the world, and student nurses today are also a diverse group, both with regard to ethnicity and age. If your practice supervisor trained in another country, they may have different expectations of what a student should be able to do, and if you are not meeting those expectations then they may view you negatively. Sometimes it may be down to a clash of personalities, especially if you have different ways of learning and working, and lastly it must be acknowledged that you may have been allocated to someone who – for reasons that are unclear – is simply not a good practice supervisor or assessor.

As we discussed earlier with Sara and Aran, it is absolutely essential that you talk to someone if your relationship with your practice supervisor or assessor is not working. If at all possible, talking to them directly is always best as sometimes it is just a case of letting them know how you are feeling and exploring solutions. Try to focus on describing how you are feeling rather than accusing them. It is quite possible that they may be really surprised and unaware that you are unhappy and will work with you to resolve the issues. However, if you cannot resolve the problems or really feel you cannot talk with them, then contact your link lecturer or personal tutor for help. Keeping quiet and saying nothing means that you will have a poor learning experience, which could adversely impact on your progression, and if it is due to poor supervision then future students will be subjected to that too.

Sometimes students wait until they leave the placement before raising any concerns about their experience and detail it all in the evaluation of their placement. This is unfair on the staff and the placement as they have not had a chance to respond to the issues you have raised. Honest evaluations are important, however, and we will finish the chapter by looking at them.

# Evaluating your placement

Evaluating your placement when you return to university at the end of a placement is essential. It is a professional expectation, with *The Code* identifying the importance of providing 'honest, accurate and constructive feedback to colleagues' (NMC, 2018a, p10). It is also an NMC requirement that universities provide students with the opportunity to give feedback; this includes the support and supervision you had while on placement (NMC, 2018b). Feedback is essential if the staff in practice are to make improvements that will benefit future students and contribute to their success on placement. Equally, feedback provides an opportunity for good practices to be identified and shared, which can enhance the learning for other students across multiple placement areas, so always try to include the particular strengths or the opportunities you found valuable on your placement.

Each university will have different types of evaluation forms, but most will include tick boxes/rating scales along with open questions. Open questions provide qualitative data, which are important for the university and the placement as they help them to understand the answers you have given. Try to give specific examples of what was good or worked well and what was not so good for you and explain why it was good or not good. If possible, provide ideas of ways you think would have made it better. If you identified any problems, did you tell anyone or do anything about it, and did this resolve the problem?

Clinical staff in practice appreciate the feedback provided by students just as you do for your assignments. So, when asked to complete an evaluation form, consider how you would feel if you didn't receive any feedback on your performance in practice or on your assignments at university, and take the time to give a fair, balanced and honest evaluation of your experience.

## Chapter summary

This chapter has explored how you can get the most out of your placement. A central theme throughout has been the importance of communicating with the staff in your placement in order to identify your learning needs, alert others when learning needs are not being met, and solve problems when difficulties arise. Patients have been identified as an important resource for learning, as well as working with other health and social care professionals in order to develop an understanding of interprofessional and multidisciplinary working. Spoke and outreach placements offer an opportunity to understand the patient journey and experience how care is integrated across different settings. While most placements will run smoothly, problems can arise. These require the student to communicate their concerns in order that the problems can be explored and resolved. However, most important of all is your willingness to engage in the learning process; this will ensure you get the most out of your placement.

# Activities: brief outline answers

## Activity 5.2   Team working (p81)

This list is not conclusive, but you may have identified some of the following: art therapists, chiropodists, dieticians, doctors, GPs, HCAs, hospital play staff, midwives, nursing associates, nursery nurses, newborn hearing screeners, occupational therapists, paramedics, pharmacists, physiotherapists, psychiatrists, psychologists, radiographers, social workers, speech and language therapists, and teachers.

## Activity 5.3   Communication (p83)

Dev introduced himself and explained who he was. He gained her permission to call her by her first name. He was aware of his body language and used the acronym SOLER to help him: by **S**itting squarely, with an **O**pen posture, **L**eaning forward slightly, and maintaining **E**ye contact; in doing so, he tried to appear **R**elaxed.

## Activity 5.5   Communication (p90)

Problems you'd find difficult to share will be personal to you, but depending on the problem people you may seek help from are friends or family, peers on the course, your personal tutor, the link tutor, student advisory services, the disability team, and your GP.

## Activity 5.6   Critical thinking (p93)

Time goes by very fast on a placement, so raising a concern early on is important. Aran should have approached the manager or lead in the placement to ask for another practice supervisor and assessor to be allocated to him as soon as he was aware that his original ones were not going to be around. If Aran had found it difficult to approach the manager, then his next action should have been to contact someone from the university. This could be the link lecturer or nominated person for the placement or his academic assessor. When a student is concerned about their learning experience, early contact with the link lecturer or equivalent is important in alerting them to a potential problem. This can take place by phone or by email, asking them if you can talk on the phone or meet up to discuss the concerns you have.

# Further reading

**Guest, M.** (2016) How to introduce yourself to patients. *Nursing Standard*, 30(41): 36–8.

Useful tips on introducing yourself to patients.

**Royal College of Nursing (RCN)** (2017) *Helping Students Get the Best from Their Practice Placements.* Available at: www.rcn.org.uk/professional-development/publications/pub-006035

A useful guide on getting the most out of your placement from preparation before evaluating afterwards.

**Sharples, K.** (2011) *Successful Practice Learning for Nursing Students*, 2nd edn. Exeter: Learning Matters.

Chapter 8, 'Succeeding in Practice', looks at the importance of motivation in learning on placement.

# Useful websites

Great Ormond Street: Real Stories

**www.gosh.nhs.uk/medical-information/real-stories**

This provides insights into children's experiences of their illness and treatments.

Health Careers: Explore Roles

**www.healthcareers.nhs.uk/explore-roles**

A useful insight into a wide range of different healthcare roles in the NHS.

UK Student Nurse Blog

**https://nursingsecrets.co.uk**

A blog site by a second-year student nurse that also includes videos. Contains some useful tips around placements.

# Chapter 6  The assessment process

Karen Elcock

---

## NMC Standards of Proficiency for Registered Nurses

This chapter will address the following platforms and proficiencies:

**Platform 1: Being an accountable professional**

Registered nurses act in the best interests of people, putting them first and providing nursing care that is person-centred, safe and compassionate. They act professionally at all times and use their knowledge and experience to make evidence-based decisions about care. They communicate effectively, are role models for others, and are accountable for their actions. Registered nurses continually reflect on their practice and keep abreast of new and emerging developments in nursing, health and care.

At the point of registration, the registered nurse will be able to:

1.1 understand and act in accordance with *The Code: Professional Standards of Practice and Behaviour for Nurses, Midwives and Nursing Associates*, and fulfil all registration requirements.

1.5 understand the demands of professional practice and demonstrate how to recognise signs of vulnerability in themselves or their colleagues and the action required to minimise risks to health.

1.8 demonstrate the knowledge, skills and ability to think critically when applying evidence and drawing on experience to make evidence informed decisions in all situations.

1.10 demonstrate resilience and emotional intelligence and be capable of explaining the rationale that influences their judgements and decisions in routine, complex and challenging situations.

1.16 demonstrate the ability to keep complete, clear, accurate and timely records.

1.17 take responsibility for continuous self-reflection, seeking and responding to support and feedback to develop their professional knowledge and skills.

## Chapter aims

After reading this chapter, you will be able to:

- explain why assessment in practice is such an important part of your course, and appreciate your responsibility in the assessment process;
- demonstrate an understanding of the terminology commonly used in the Practice Assessment Documents;
- explain the importance of the initial and midpoint interviews;
- demonstrate how to identify your learning needs and write SMART learning objectives;
- demonstrate how to receive and respond to feedback from your practice supervisors and assessors in a professional manner;
- recognise when it is appropriate to seek support and help when you are having difficulties with the assessment process; and
- identify the learning that you can take from one placement to the next.

# Introduction

The assessment process is an essential part of placement learning, providing you with a structured approach to learning and feedback on your progress, as well as identifying areas for further development both during and at the end of the placement. It is also the aspect that many students can find very stressful as failure in practice can impact on further progression on the programme. This chapter will therefore discuss why assessment in practice is so important – its value to you in developing your skills, knowledge and professional attitudes – and will explore your own responsibility in the assessment process, as well as those in practice and at the university. Each step of the assessment process will be explored, from the initial interview to the midpoint interview, through to the all-important final interview. Underpinning these stages in the assessment process is the Practice Assessment Document, which we will refer to as a PAD throughout this chapter. Other terminology commonly used in the assessment process, such as skills, knowledge, attitudes and proficiencies, will be explained to enable you to construct SMART learning objectives that will enable you to plan and measure your learning more effectively. The practice assessment process can feel far more personal than formal assignments at university due to the relationship built up over the length of the placement with your practice supervisor and assessor. As feedback is given face-to-face, it is sometimes difficult to separate judgements that are made about your performance as a student nurse from the feeling that they are made about you as a person. Therefore, guidance on receiving and responding to feedback from your practice supervisors and assessors will be discussed, particularly when the feedback identifies areas for improvement or indicates potential for failing elements in the document.

The importance of seeking support and help early when there is the potential for failure or when you are having difficulties will be discussed to ensure appropriate action plans are developed and implemented that can enable a positive outcome. The chapter will close with suggestions on how you can use what you have learnt, as well as use the feedback received from one placement to inform your learning in the next placement.

# The value of assessment in practice

As a student nurse, you will be assessed throughout your course on both theory and practice, and you will need to pass both in order to register as a nurse. However, the practice element can often be seen as more challenging as the parameters are far more difficult to control compared to an academic assignment. Assignments have well-defined guidelines with a clear brief of what is required, a pre-planned submission date that does not change, and are usually assessed by a team of staff familiar to you. The practice assessment, however, is not so clear-cut. Practice is unpredictable, making planning more difficult. In addition, there are competing demands, with the needs of patients and service users taking priority over your needs to have assessment elements completed. This means that meetings to review progress or sign off proficiencies may have to be changed, making the assessment process more difficult to complete.

It is the duration of time over which you are assessed, however, that makes the practice assessment both so different and so important. While not ideal, many students will find themselves at some point staying up all night finishing an assignment or cramming for an exam. For theory, you are assessed on the final assignment you submit, not on the work/drafts you have written along the way. For assessment in practice, you are being judged over the length of the placement (often called continuous assessment), so you have to be consistent in your performance throughout. You cannot take a laid-back approach during your placement and then put all your effort into the last few days, just as you cannot provide below-par or 'just about OK' care to the people you are caring for. The care you deliver must be of a high standard at all times, both as a student and as a registered nurse. However, it is recognised that you are learning to become a nurse, and so will not be fully confident or proficient in everything you do straight away, but during your time in practice you will learn to become both confident and proficient as you learn new skills and practise them. The *Standards of Proficiency* published by the NMC (2018e) identify the proficiencies (knowledge, skills and behaviours) you are required to demonstrate in order to register and practise as a nurse by the end of your programme. Your PAD will have been designed to enable you to be assessed on many of these proficiencies and on the skills listed in Annexe A and Annexe B, which can be found at the end of these standards. While your theoretical assignments will assess your knowledge and application of theory to practice (e.g. through case studies, scenarios and OSCAs), it is in practice that your application of the knowledge taught in university to the real world of practice will be assessed. In addition, this assessment will also focus on your clinical skills and the manner (behaviour) in which you carry them out. Let's look at these three areas of knowledge, skills and behaviour in a little more detail in order that you understand what you are being assessed on by your practice assessor.

# Knowledge, skills and behaviour

Knowledge relates to the theory and facts, often called 'know-that'. You will acquire knowledge through your classes but also through your reading and research and through your life experiences. As we discussed earlier in this book, your course cannot teach you everything. This means that on each placement, you will come across situations where you have had the theory that relates to the activities or interventions you are involved in, but there will also be situations where you have not. Sometimes you may be taught about them later in the course, but for some situations that are less common you may never be taught about them within your course. This means that it is important to undertake further reading and research around your experiences in practice in order to fully understand what you are doing and why.

Skills are the practical application of knowledge, the 'know-how'. Nursing skills include the very practical skills such as taking observations and giving medications but also encompass skills such as communication and, later in your course, your leadership and supervision skills. Again, sometimes you will have been taught skills at university that you will then use in practice so will be able to demonstrate you 'know how' to do something, and sometimes you will be faced with learning new skills in practice and so develop your 'know-how' through the real world of practice. It is likely that you will focus on learning *how* to undertake the wide range of skills that are required to be a nurse. This is understandable as it will enable you to feel like a nurse and so feel part of the team. However, it is important to remember that in order to demonstrate that you are capable of safe and effective practice, you will need to be able to demonstrate that not only do you know *how* to perform a skill, but also that you know *why*. The following case study provides an example of a student who 'knows how' but does not 'know why'.

## Case study: Toni

Toni is on her first placement. Her practice supervisor shows her how to undertake urinalysis. By the end of her first week, she is really competent at this skill; she knows how to test urine and record the findings accurately. However, she has never asked the reason for doing it and her practice supervisor has never told her, so she has the 'know-how' but not the 'know-that' or 'know-why'.

## Activity 6.1   Reflection

Have you ever been in a situation where you have been asked to undertake skills or activities that you didn't fully understand the reason for or why they needed to be completed?

If your answer is 'yes', what should you have done in the situation?

*An outline answer to this activity is given at the end of the chapter.*

There will be occasions when it is not appropriate to ask why you have been asked to do something (e.g. in an emergency situation where a delay could put people at risk), but wherever possible in a situation such as that, or when it is busy, ask if you can debrief later to discuss what happened and why the different interventions were undertaken.

Behaviour is the third component that will be assessed by your practice supervisors and assessors, and it will be assessed throughout your placements. Behaviours are also called attitudes or attributes, and describe the manner in which you behave as a nursing student and the way that you carry out care interventions. Consider Activity 6.2.

## Activity 6.2   Critical thinking

List some of the behaviours you think that a practice assessor would be looking at when assessing you in practice.

*An outline answer to this activity is given at the end of the chapter.*

The behaviours that you are assessed on are not just about your ability to demonstrate care and compassion, but also around professional behaviours. It is likely that your PAD will include professional values that you will be assessed on. In England, all universities have adopted the same document format, and this includes a list of professional values that you are assessed on for each placement. The professional values identify the types of behaviours expected of you and relate to the 6Cs and the four themes in *The Code* (NMC, 2018a). Table 6.1 lists the professional values students are assessed on in the first part of their programme.

| Prioritise people |
|---|
| 1. The student maintains confidentiality in accordance with *The Code*. |
| 2. The student is non-judgemental, respectful and courteous at all times when interacting with patients/service users/carers and all colleagues. |
| 3. The student maintains the person's privacy and dignity, seeks consent prior to care, and advocates on their behalf. |
| 4. The student is caring, compassionate and sensitive to the needs of others. |
| 5. The student understands their professional responsibility in adopting and promoting a healthy lifestyle for the well-being of themselves and others. |

| Practise effectively |
|---|
| 6. The student maintains consistent, safe and person-centred practice. |
| 7. The student is able to work effectively within the interdisciplinary team with the intent of building professional relationships. |
| 8. The student makes a consistent effort to engage in the requisite standards of care and learning based on best available evidence. |

| Preserve safety |
|---|
| 9. The student demonstrates openness (candour), trustworthiness and integrity. |
| 10. The student reports any concerns to the appropriate professional member of staff when appropriate (e.g. safeguarding). |
| 11. The student demonstrates the ability to listen, seek clarification and carry out instructions safely. |
| 12. The student is able to recognise and work within the limitations of their own knowledge, skills and professional boundaries, and understand that they are responsible for their own actions. |

| Promote professionalism and trust |
|---|
| 13. The student's personal presentation and dress code is in accordance with the local policy. |
| 14. The student maintains an appropriate professional attitude regarding punctuality and communicates appropriately if unable to attend placement. |
| 15. The student demonstrates that they are self-aware and can recognise their own emotions and those of others in different situations. |

*Table 6.1*  Professional values

*Source*: PLPLG (2019)

While knowledge, skills and behaviour have been discussed separately, when observing you in practice your practice assessor will be assessing how you integrate all three elements in care delivery. Look at the case study describing Tracey's performance caring for a child and then answer the questions in Activity 6.3.

## Case study: Tracey

Tracey is on a paediatric placement and is taking observations on a 5-year-old child who has returned from surgery that day. Her practice supervisor, Rosi, who she is working with that day, notices that Tracey checks that she has the correct cuff size and takes the observations and records them accurately; however, she says very little to the child while she is doing the observations and ignores the parents completely. Later in the day, Rosi discusses how Tracey managed the care of the child she had been caring for all shift. Tracey is able to tell her what the normal parameters are for a 5-year-old child and explains the rationale for taking observations and why it was so important to ensure she had the correct cuff size. Rosi asks why she didn't talk to the family when taking the observations. Tracey says that they made her very nervous as they were watching her so closely and she was focusing on completing the observations correctly.

## Activity 6.3   Critical thinking

How well do you think Tracey has done in demonstrating her knowledge, skills and attitudes with regard to the post-operative observations she carried out?

Which of the professional values in Table 6.1 may she have not fully met?

*An outline answer to this activity is given at the end of the chapter.*

As you gain experience and progress through your programme, your knowledge and understanding will grow, and you will develop increasing confidence and competence in performing practical skills and acquire the professional behaviours required. An essential professional behaviour expected of you is your engagement in learning and demonstrating this by taking an active role in seeking learning opportunities and seeking feedback.

# The assessment process

The PAD has four stages that need to be completed for each placement: the orientation to the placement, followed by the assessment process, which has three distinct parts to it. You will find these three stages are clearly set out in your PAD, and cover the initial interview, the interim interview and the final interview (Figure 6.1). Within the PAD will also be the proficiencies and other elements that you are assessed on and must pass by the end of the part.

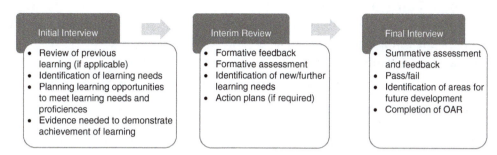

*Figure 6.1* The assessment process

While the assessment process has three formal parts to it, it is actually a continuous process that involves your practice supervisor planning learning opportunities, working with you, and observing your performance and providing feedback. Your practice assessor will work with you at key points, and use observation, questioning and collation of feedback from others to inform their assessment of your progress and achievement. The assessment process should involve opportunities for regular formative feedback so that you know how you are progressing, and identifies your strengths and areas for improvement or identification of new areas to focus on to further develop your knowledge and skills. Formative feedback offers you an opportunity to make improvements (where required) before the final summative assessment. Summative feedback occurs at the end of your placement and is the point at which a decision is made as to whether you have met all the requirements for that placement or not, and so forms part of the summative assessment.

# The initial interview

You should have had an orientation to the placement area on your first day that covers health and safety (e.g. resuscitation equipment, fire exits, local policies), responding to emergencies, shifts, and so on. The initial interview focuses on your learning and is essential if your learning activities in practice are going to be structured to meet your learning needs and enable you to achieve the required elements in your PAD. It should take place within the first 48 hours of commencing your placement. This meeting offers you a chance to get to know your practice supervisor and assessor, and should cover the following key areas:

- the learning opportunities available to you on the placement;
- any learning needs identified from previous placements;

- areas you wish to focus on;
- the elements in the PAD that can be achieved on this placement, and so what you will be assessed on;
- an agreed plan of the skills and learning opportunities for you to focus on based on the above during the placement;
- the type of evidence you need to gather to demonstrate your achievement of your identified learning needs/proficiencies; and
- the date for your interim interview.

# The interim interview

This should take place roughly halfway through your placement so is often called the midpoint interview. It will take place either with your practice supervisor or your practice assessor, depending on your university's requirements; if it is the practice assessor, then ideally your practice supervisor should attend. This interview should not be the first time you meet to discuss your progress (unless you are on a very short placement), but it is a formal stage in the assessment process where you should receive feedback about the progress you are making.

Before the interim meeting, you should reflect on your progress so far. Consider your strengths and areas for improvement with regard to your knowledge, skills and behaviours, as well as any areas you wish to particularly focus on in the second half of your placement. You will receive feedback from your practice assessor on your strengths, and any areas for improvement should be identified and discussed. Any elements you have achieved in your PAD so far may be signed off at this stage (although they can also be signed off as you go along). In England, the interim interview also includes an interim review of your progress in meeting the professional values and identifies any aspects that you need to improve upon (if any). The most common concerns around professional values identified about students at the midpoint are around timekeeping and engagement in learning. Consider the following case study, which focuses on an interim interview, and then answer the questions in Activity 6.4.

---

## Case study: Sasha

Sasha is in her first placement in the final year of her nursing programme and halfway through an eight-week placement on an acute inpatient ward. She is finding that there is a lot of new information to learn and does not feel confident in all the skills she is expected to demonstrate, especially around delegating care to the healthcare assistants, which means she rushes round trying to do everything herself.

This has not been helped by comments from staff, which have shown that they have an increased expectation of her skills and knowledge as a final-year student. She has been working with her allocated practice supervisor for the past couple of days and has a meeting planned with them and her practice assessor to discuss her progress.

## Activity 6.4    Critical thinking

How do you think Sasha should prepare, and what should she say?

What do you think her practice assessor might feed back?

Who might help her in this scenario?

*An outline answer to this activity is given at the end of the chapter.*

If there are concerns about any aspect of your performance, an action plan may be developed. This can take place at any point in the assessment process where concerns arise regarding your progress or performance, but they are commonly developed at the interim interview.

# The action plan

Students can find discussion of an action plan very threatening, but should see this as a positive activity, as an action plan ensures that there is an agreed strategy to assist them to succeed rather than allowing them to continue to muddle through and potentially fail at the end of the placement. The headings in an action plan may vary in different countries across the UK but are likely to cover:

- the nature of the concerns identified about the student's performance (this may be knowledge, skills or behaviours, or a mix of all three);
- what the student needs to demonstrate to show improvements in the areas identified;
- the support that will be provided, and by whom, to help the student to achieve; and
- a date for review of progress and summary of the progress made.

Table 6.2 provides an example of an action plan used in response to the concerns raised about Sasha in the case study earlier (for more details, see also the outline answer for Activity 6.4 at the end of the chapter).

| Nature of concern<br>Refer to professional value(s), proficiency and/or episode of care (Specific) | What does the student need to demonstrate?<br>*Objectives and measure of success* (Measurable, Achievable and Realistic) | Support available and who is responsible | Date for review<br>(Timed) | Review/feedback |
|---|---|---|---|---|
| Sasha fails to delegate aspects of care to others, and consequently essential care activities such as observations and preparation of patients for discharge are not being completed on time.<br>Professional value 9<br>Proficiency 19 | Sasha will plan her priorities at the start of each shift and identify which activities should be delegated to the staff in the team she is working with. She will check progress by her team at regular intervals during the shift to ensure the essential activities are being completed on time.<br>If care is being delayed, she will inform her practice supervisor or the staff member in charge of the shift and seek advice and help. | Sasha will discuss her plan with her practice supervisor at the start of each shift and provide an update on progress midway through the shift.<br>Advised to talk with her personal tutor for resources she can access on delegation. | Review progress after two weeks. | **Date:** dd/mm/yyyy<br><br>**Comments:**<br>Sasha has written a plan at the start of each shift and her work is now more organised. She has found delegating to some staff difficult and we have discussed how she might develop her assertiveness skills. |

*Table 6.2* Action plan

*Source*: PLPLG (2019)

# The final interview and the Ongoing Achievement Record

The final (summative) interview should take place at the end of the placement. This will cover all the same elements as in the interim interview above with any additional learning needs/improvements identified that need to be taken forward to your next placement. If you have been recorded as failing any elements within your PAD, your university will have a process to manage this (e.g. retaking failed elements on your next placement or undertaking a retrieval placement to be assessed on the failed elements). Additional support will be put in place to support you through this process.

The Ongoing Achievement Record (OAR) is also completed at the end of your placement by your practice assessor and is a summary of your strengths and areas for development as detailed in your PAD. The OAR is a continuous record and summary of your strengths and areas for development from each placement across the programme. At the end of each part of your programme, your practice assessor and academic assessor will sign to confirm whether you have fulfilled all the requirements within the PAD for that part.

The assessment process has discussed a number of activities (e.g. identifying learning needs and feedback that need to take place in order to plan your learning), and we will now look at these in more detail, as well as exploring writing SMART objectives to help with both of these activities.

# How to identify your learning needs

There are a number of strategies and tools to help you identify your learning needs; each one requires you to dedicate some time to identifying them. However, this will be time well spent as it will enable you to be clear as to what your aims and learning needs are for each of your placements. Forward planning will also assist your practice supervisor in planning the learning opportunities you will need to achieve the proficiencies within your PAD and any additional learning needs you have identified.

## Previous feedback

If you have already had a placement, then a good starting point is your PAD and your Ongoing Achievement Record (OAR), both of which will contain feedback from your previous placement(s). If this is your first placement, then you may have received feedback on your performance in undertaking skills at university that you can use to identify your initial goals. For example, you may need more practice at certain skills or need to develop more confidence in talking to patients or service users. In addition to looking back, your PAD can also help you to look forward in identifying future learning needs. You were asked to do this in Activity 5.1 in Chapter 5, so it is worth looking at this activity again.

Your PAD sets out the proficiencies and other learning activities you need to achieve on your placement. Some will be achievable on any placement and some may be easier on specific types of placements, particularly around some more complex physical health skills or therapeutic interventions. It is therefore essential to identify those that may only be achieved on your current placement and make those a higher priority than those that can be achieved on any another placement. Your practice supervisor will help you identify which proficiencies can be achieved. One way of helping you to identify your learning needs and consider how they can be met is by using a SWOT or SLOT analysis.

## SWOT or SLOT analysis

You may already be familiar with a SWOT analysis (**S**trengths, **W**eaknesses, **O**pportunities and **T**hreats). A SLOT analysis is essentially the same but replaces the 'W' with an 'L', which stands for **L**earning needs, and is a far more positive way at looking at what it is you need to learn or achieve on your placement. It is possible that some weaknesses could be placed under threats. For example, if you lack confidence, this could be a threat in enabling you to get involved and participate in learning opportunities. Figure 6.2 describes these elements further. Now complete Activity 6.5, which applies the use of a SWOT/ SLOT analysis to your learning needs identified in your PAD.

| Strengths | Weaknesses or Learning needs |
|---|---|
| What you are good at. Consider what you have learnt, including theory and clinical skills, as well as your interpersonal skills. | Areas that you are not good at/don't know/have no experience of, and so need to learn about/improve upon. |
| **Opportunities** | **Threats** |
| Opportunities/resources that are available in practice to help you achieve your learning needs. Includes people and activities/experiences available. | What might prevent you from achieving your learning needs (e.g. time, support available, own confidence). |

*Figure 6.2* A SWOT/SLOT analysis

## Activity 6.5   Critical thinking

Look at your previous PAD and your OAR to help you draw up a list of areas that were identified as knowledge, skills or behaviours that you need to develop.

If you haven't started practice yet, then identify areas within your PAD that you want/need to focus on in your first placement.

Use the areas identified to help you complete a SWOT/SLOT analysis that you can take to practice with you.

*As this activity is based on your own learning needs, there is no outline answer at the end of the chapter.*

Once you have identified what you want to learn, it can be helpful to turn these wants and needs into clearly measurable objectives.

# Writing SMART learning objectives

SMART objectives are valuable as they provide a very clear focus on what you are going to do by when, and how you will know when you have achieved it. A SMART goal must be:

- *Specific*: Be precise about what it is that you want to be able to do.
- *Measurable*: Consider how much, how many, and how you will know you have achieved your objective. What will you need to be able to do to demonstrate achievement?

- *Achievable*: Are there sufficient opportunities to practise/achieve your objective? Is there sufficient time available?
- *Relevant*: Is the objective relevant to your learning needs?
- *Time-bound/timely*: Do your objectives have a clear timeline of what needs to be done by when? Have interim review dates been set?

If your objectives are not SMART, then you may find you don't achieve what you or your practice supervisors or assessors expect. Take the case of Maria.

---

## Case study: Maria

Maria has started on her first placement and meets with her practice supervisor, Jack, to discuss her PAD and what she aims to achieve on her placement. She has pre-prepared what she wants to focus on and explains that she wants to further develop the core skills she learnt in the skills and simulation suite at university (strengths). She identifies these as taking observations, handwashing and fluid balance. She says she needs help with fluid balance as she gets nervous with numbers (weakness/learning need). Her practice supervisor tells her that these are good choices as all the patients need observations taken every day, many are on fluid balance charts, and hand hygiene is an essential skill on any placement (opportunities). Jack tells Maria that her lack of confidence with numeracy skills (threat) is not uncommon in nursing students, and lots of practice on placement will help her gain confidence.

Three weeks later, they sit down to review how she is doing, and it is clear that Maria has not made the expected progress in achieving her identified learning needs. She has been practising the skills she identified, but Jack had expected her to also have a greater understanding of what she is doing and why.

---

Maria had started her placement well, coming prepared with what she wanted to learn, but the lack of clear steps on how she was going to achieve her learning needs meant there was no real plan in place for her to succeed. What Maria needed were SMART objectives. Complete Activity 6.6 to identify these for Maria.

## Activity 6.6   Critical thinking

Write SMART objectives for Maria's learning needs to be able to record fluid balance and demonstrate her numeracy skills.

*An outline answer to this activity is given at the end of the chapter.*

If you have SMART objectives, it is far easier to understand exactly what you are aiming for and what your practice supervisor is expecting you to be doing, both in undertaking care activities in practice and any additional background reading so that you can provide the theory to support your practice. This also means that feedback can be more specifically targeted on how you met those SMART objectives. However, it will be impossible to write SMART objectives for every activity you undertake in practice as you would spend your whole placement writing them out. SMART objectives are useful for focusing on specific areas you wish to work on and when areas for improvement have been identified (see Table 6.2, which uses SMART objectives). It is in the identifying of areas for improvement that feedback becomes particularly important.

# Receiving and responding to feedback

Feedback is essential to enable you to understand what you are doing well and where you need to improve. Feedback can be either positive or negative, or a mixture of both. Positive feedback identifies what you are doing well, whereas negative feedback identifies areas in which you are not doing well. If handled in a constructive way, both forms of feedback are valuable to you. Duffy (2013) explores the definition of 'constructive' and identifies keywords linked with constructive feedback as 'helpful', 'practical', 'productive', 'useful' and 'valuable' (p51). Activity 6.7 will help you to understand different levels of feedback.

## Activity 6.7 Critical thinking

Consider the following feedback statements:

1. You have done well today.
2. You completed that wound dressing well.
3. You completed that drug round well today, but you need to read up on the common drugs used on this placement so that you understand what they are for and their common side effects.

How helpful would you find each of these feedback statements?

*An outline answer to this activity is given at the end of the chapter.*

So, feedback is not just about saying you have done well. Feedback that is constructive explains why and how you did well and offers ideas and guidance on any areas for improvement.

It is important to remember that you have a responsibility when it comes to feedback. Don't wait for feedback to be given to you; instead, actively seek feedback from the colleagues you work with. While your practice supervisor and assessor will be the key people to approach for feedback, you should also seek feedback from the wide range of health and social care professionals you work with. Each of these have a professional responsibility to support and develop learners, so should be able to give you feedback if they have been working alongside you. There should be sections in your PAD where they provide written feedback on your performance. By seeking feedback from different members of the team you are working with, you will receive different perspectives on your performance, which can be invaluable in gaining a rounded picture of how you are progressing. Don't forget to also seek feedback from unqualified staff, who can provide feedback on your team working and your approach to delegating care activities to them.

In order to get feedback that is helpful you need to ask the right questions. If you ask for feedback by saying, 'How am I doing?' this is very vague and is likely to lead to responses that may be equally vague such as, 'You're doing well', or can open you up to receiving a whole host of feedback that is not valuable or could be destructive. Asking a question such as, 'Can you tell me what I am doing well and areas I need to improve on?' will be more helpful, but it is a big question given the range of care activities you will have been involved in and may lead to responses that are still not specific enough to be helpful. To get very specific feedback, focus on what it is you want to know. For example, if you had identified medication management as an area to work on in your meetings with your practice supervisor or assessor, then ask, 'Can you tell me what I did well on the drug round today and what areas I need to improve on with regard to medication management?' This helps the person you are seeking feedback from to focus their comments so that it relates to the specific skill, behaviour or knowledge that you have been working on.

## Feedback from service users

In addition to the nurses and other health and social care professionals you meet on placement, you will also be expected to seek feedback from service users about how they perceived your approach to care delivery with them and how it may have impacted on them. The case study about Alison provides an example of service user feedback. Consider your own experience so far on your course and then answer Activity 6.8.

### Case study: Alison

Alison is on placement and has been working with her practice supervisor. It is incredibly busy. Yesterday she was given a group of patients to care for. The next day, her practice supervisor suggests that it would be helpful to get some feedback from the patients she cared for that can be recorded in her PAD. One of the patients,

*(Continued)*

(Continued)

Mrs Amblin, says that she found Alison really friendly and kind, but adds that yesterday Alison left her with a bowl and said she'd come back to help her wash any areas she couldn't do for herself. Unfortunately, Alison got caught up with another patient, and when she got back Mrs Amblin was sat half-washed with a very cold bowl of water. Mrs Amblin suggests to Alison that in future if the areas she couldn't manage were done first, then she could finish washing the rest of herself; that way, she would not then be sitting and waiting half-washed. Alison thinks this is a brilliant idea and decides this will be the way she approaches all her patients in future.

## Activity 6.8   Critical thinking

What do you think are the possible difficulties or issues in seeking feedback from patients/service users or carers?

*An outline answer to this activity is given at the end of the chapter.*

There are also benefits to seeking service user feedback, as Alison found above, which a number of studies have reported. One of these studies is summarised in the research summary below.

## Research summary: Service user feedback

Speers and Lathlean (2015) undertook a study with mental health service users, mentors (now called practice supervisors/assessors) and students. The research found that service users evaluated the process of providing feedback to students very positively, feeling it enabled them to give something back to the students as well as making the relationship more level. Students found that it had a positive impact on the dynamics of their relationships with service users and that it resulted in changes in their behaviours, with a greater self-awareness of their abilities.

The findings in the research summary are also supported by McMahon-Parkes et al. (2016), who undertook a similar study with adult field students in which mentors commented that they felt service user feedback improved students' competence and confidence. These mentors also said that they used the feedback when assessing the students' professional values and communication and interpersonal skills.

While feedback from service users is generally very positive, unfortunately sometimes the feedback you receive from staff in practice may not be. In these situations, you need to learn how to receive feedback in a measured and professional manner.

## Responding to feedback

When receiving feedback, it is important to listen very carefully to what is being said. You will be receiving feedback throughout your course, and once you qualify this will continue as a registered nurse as part of your **annual appraisal**. Learning how to accept feedback in a professional manner is therefore an essential part of your journey in becoming a registered nurse.

Feedback is provided to help you understand what you do well and to help you improve. It is easy to stop listening to what is being said if you receive feedback you were not expecting or if you don't understand what is being said to you. It is not unusual to start constructing an answer in your head in defence before someone has finished speaking. So, when receiving feedback, take a deep breath, focus on what is being said, and listen to what they have to say until they have finished. If the feedback you receive is vague or if you feel that it is inaccurate, then ask them to be more precise and give examples to help you understand. For example, if they say you are disorganised, you need to ask them for clarification without sounding defensive:

> *I'd really appreciate it if you could give some examples of when I was disorganised and offer me some advice on how I could improve.*

Sometimes you need them to be even more precise. For example:

> *You have said that I need to improve my knowledge of drugs. I understand this, but there are a lot of drugs to learn about. I'd appreciate it if you could advise which ones I should focus on during this placement.*

Receiving feedback that is not all praise is difficult, so taking time afterwards to reflect on what has been said is important. Ask if you can take some time out to assimilate what has been said. This will allow your emotions to settle and enable you to gain a more balanced perspective of what has been said. Consider if what has been said is accurate, even if it is difficult to accept. Then, when you are feeling calmer, ask if you can discuss it further when you feel more able to explore what has been said.

Feedback on your performance can feel very personal, especially if it only focuses on what you have not done well. This type of destructive feedback can have a significant effect on your self-esteem and can be very difficult to hear and then respond to without becoming defensive and emotional. Destructive feedback that fails to provide clear examples and only focuses on the negatives needs to be challenged, which can be very difficult as a student. If this happens to you, you need to seek support.

# Seeking support and help when concerns arise regarding your performance in practice

Sometimes the assessment process may not go as you would hope. If problems arise, then you need to seek help as soon as possible. There are a number of people you can seek help from, such as the link lecturer, your academic assessor or your personal tutor. These roles are discussed in more detail in Chapter 4. Involving their support early on can often prevent problems escalating, and they can ensure that the practice supervisor and assessor are also supported to support you, as well as ensuring a fair assessment takes place.

# Identify the learning that you can take from one placement to the next

At the end of each placement, you will be expected to summarise your own learning in your Practice Assessment Document, and in conjunction with your practice assessor will identify and record further learning that you need to take forward to your next placement. A summary of your strengths and areas for further development that have been identified will also be documented in your Ongoing Achievement Record. These areas can then be used to plan your learning on your next placement.

# Your responsibility in the assessment process

We have touched on this throughout this chapter but bring the key elements together here for you. In order to gain the most from each placement, it is essential that you are proactive in the assessment process. This means that you must come prepared for your placement and have some ideas about what you want and need to learn. Your PAD is central to the assessment process, so there will be an expectation that you have read through it and have an understanding of what is expected of you. Starting your placement having already identified which areas you wish to focus on in your PAD, or areas you need to develop further following feedback from previous placements, is helpful. It will assist your practice supervisor in planning your learning, provide you with some control over your learning, and show the staff you will be working with that you are interested in learning during your placement. It is essential that you have your PAD with you on each shift (if it is a paper document) or know how to access it if it is stored online as this ensures that it can be kept updated as you progress. Failure to provide your PAD when it is asked for could prevent your progression on the programme. Your OAR must also be available at the initial and final interviews.

Once you have started your placement, it is essential that you show interest in learning and actively seek learning opportunities that fit with your learning needs. You know what it is that you want/need to learn, but your practice supervisor may not always remember everything you agreed to. So, keep your ears and eyes open as to what is going on so that you can alert staff when something comes up that you have identified as a learning need or is a skill within your PAD that you need to achieve.

You also have a responsibility to actively seek out feedback from the people you work with, and not wait passively for it to be provided to you. However, consider the timing of requesting feedback. Asking when it is really busy or in front of other staff is not a good idea.

You may have noticed from the above that the words 'proactive' and 'actively' are mentioned several times in this section. Taking responsibility for your learning by not waiting for others to suggest learning activities or offer feedback, as well as getting involved in what is taking place in practice, is important as a developing professional.

## Chapter summary

This chapter has taken you through the assessment process, which is an essential part of your course as practice constitutes 50 per cent of your programme and is where significant learning takes place as you apply the theory learnt at university to the real world of practice. The assessment process involves the assessment of your knowledge, skills and behaviours in order to confirm that you have met the NMC proficiencies that are required to register as a nurse. The Practice Assessment Document sets out the knowledge, skills and professional values you are expected to achieve in each part of your programme. Your responsibility in the assessment process is centred on your active engagement with the process, from the initial interview through to the interim interview and final interview. Strategies for engaging in the assessment process have been explored, focusing on the identification of your learning needs and seeking feedback to enable you to develop insight into your strengths and areas for development that will inform future assessments.

## Activities: brief outline answers

### Activity 6.1   Reflection (p102)

If you have been asked to carry out an activity or intervention that you don't understand the rationale for, you should always ask for an explanation. If you are still unclear, make a note to look it up when you get an opportunity or to talk to your personal tutor.

### Activity 6.2   Critical thinking (p102)

There is a long list of behaviours you could choose from, but ones that you may have come up with are likely to relate to the 6Cs: care, compassion, competence, communication, courage and commitment.

## Activity 6.3    Critical thinking (p104)

Tracey demonstrated good knowledge and understanding of observations. She performed the skill competently. However, her communication skills were poor (professional value 2). The skill of taking observations is not just about competence in performing the skill, but also includes gaining consent (professional value 3) and explaining to the child and the child's family what she is going to do (professional value 2); in other words, it is also about her behaviour/manner in carrying out the skill.

## Activity 6.4    Critical thinking (p107)

When preparing for an interim or final interview, it would be useful for Sasha to make a list of the different skills and activities that she has been doing and identify what she thinks she does well and what areas she feels less confident about.

Ideally, her practice assessor will pick up on the same strengths and areas for development that Sasha has, but sometimes areas the student has not considered or realised are identified (good and less good). With regard to delegation, she should highlight the proficiencies and professional values related to delegation and team working.

If a student is aware that there may be some difficult conversations during an interim or final interview, they can request the support of their academic assessor/personal tutor or link lecturer. Equally, a practice assessor who has concerns about a student's progress should raise them with the academic assessor as soon as possible to ensure that appropriate support is in place.

## Activity 6.6    Critical thinking (p111)

There are two key objectives for Maria. The first relates to demonstrating her skill at recording fluid balance for patients and the second relates to the knowledge underpinning this skill.

Each shift Maria is on duty, she will record the fluid balances for all patients in A Bay who have a fluid chart, which will be checked by her practice supervisor at the end of each shift and feedback given to Maria on the accuracy of her recording.

By the end of the second week, Maria will be able to:

- record fluid intake and output accurately for the patients in A Bay on their fluid charts, which will be confirmed by her practice supervisor;
- explain whether each patient is in a positive or negative balance at the end of the shift;
- explain why recording fluid balance is important for each of the patients with a fluid chart; and
- explain the signs and symptoms of dehydration and fluid retention.

## Activity 6.7    Critical thinking (p112)

1.  This is likely to make you feel good, but does it mean you did well at everything or generally did well, or simply worked hard?

2.  This is helpful as you know that this is specifically about wound care, but were you perfect or are there areas you could improve further, and if so what?

3.  This is far more specific, but you may need to ask what the common drugs are you should focus on.

## Activity 6.8    Critical thinking (p114)

One of the main difficulties in requesting feedback from a patient/service user or carer is that they can feel vulnerable and may believe that any criticisms they give could impact on the care they receive, so the feedback given only focuses on the positives. It is also possible that not all would have the knowledge and skills to provide feedback that has value and is meaningful to students.

# Further reading

**Duffy, K.** (2013) Providing constructive feedback to students during mentoring. *Nursing Standard*, 27(31): 50–6.

A useful insight into the feedback process.

**Royal College of Nursing (RCN)** (2017) *Helping Students Get the Best from Their Practice Placements.* Available at: www.rcn.org.uk/professional-development/publications/pub-006035

Although this refers to mentors, this has a useful table that takes you through the assessment process.

# Useful websites

Pan London Practice Learning Group

**https://plplg.uk**

An excellent website primarily aimed at practice supervisors and assessors, but it has useful resources to help you understand the assessment process.

Supporting Information on Standards for Student Supervision and Assessment

**www.nmc.org.uk/supporting-information-on-standards-for-student-supervision-and-assessment/**

An NMC web page that provides information on the different roles involved in student supervision and assessment. The section on student empowerment is particularly useful.

# Chapter 7 Planning your elective

Michelle McBride

---

## NMC Standards of Proficiency for Registered Nurses

This chapter will address the following platforms and proficiencies:

### Platform 1: Being an accountable professional

Registered nurses act in the best interests of people, putting them first and providing nursing care that is person-centred, safe and compassionate. They act professionally at all times and use their knowledge and experience to make evidence-based decisions about care. They communicate effectively, are role models for others, and are accountable for their actions. Registered nurses continually reflect on their practice and keep abreast of new and emerging developments in nursing, health and care.

At the point of registration, the registered nurse will be able to:

1.5 understand the demands of professional practice and demonstrate how to recognise signs of vulnerability in themselves or their colleagues and the action required to minimise risks to health.

### Platform 2: Promoting health and preventing ill health

Registered nurses play a key role in improving and maintaining the mental, physical and behavioural health and wellbeing of people, families, communities and populations. They support and enable people at all stages of life and in all care settings to make informed choices about how to manage health challenges in order to maximise their quality of life and improve health outcomes. They are actively involved in the prevention of and protection against disease and ill health and engage in public health, community development and global health agendas, and in the reduction of health inequalities.

At the point of registration, the registered nurse will be able to:

2.2 demonstrate knowledge of epidemiology, demography, genomics and the wider determinants of health, illness and wellbeing and apply this to an understanding of global patterns of health and wellbeing outcomes.

**Platform 6: Improving safety and quality of care**

Registered nurses make a key contribution to the continuous monitoring and quality improvement of care and treatment in order to enhance health outcomes and people's experience of nursing and related care. They assess risks to safety or experience and take appropriate action to manage those, putting the best interests, needs and preferences of people first.

At the point of registration, the registered nurse will be able to:

6.1   understand and apply the principles of health and safety legislation and regulations and maintain safe work and care environments.

6.5   demonstrate the ability to accurately undertake risk assessments in a range of care settings, using a range of contemporary assessment and improvement tools.

## Chapter aims

After reading this chapter, you will be able to:

- identify the benefits and potential learning when undertaking an elective placement;
- understand the process of planning for an elective and how to minimise risk;
- recognise what being 'culturally sensitive' means and how to develop this; and
- discuss how undertaking an elective placement can enhance personal and professional development.

# Introduction

The chance to undertake an elective placement as part of a pre-registration nursing course is now commonly available to students within the UK (RCN, 2018b). An elective is an opportunity for a student to choose a placement/clinical experience they wish to gain experience in, which is in addition to the placements with local placement providers scheduled by the university. Elective placements are planned into the curriculum at a set time in the programme and contribute towards practice hours. International placements, in particular, are now offered at many institutions, and offer an opportunity for nursing students to achieve many new personal and professional skills and competencies that they would not have the opportunity to achieve within the UK. The World Health Organization estimates that of the 43.5 million health workers globally, 20.7 million are nurses and midwives, illustrating that there is a wealth of opportunities awaiting student nurses across the globe; the challenge is to find them, access them and plan a meaningful experience

(WHO, 2016). A nursing elective can be a once-in-a-lifetime opportunity. Whether you're an adult, child, mental health or learning disability nurse, you will have the opportunity to experience new clinical environments, compare similarities and differences in how healthcare professionals deliver care in other countries, and in some countries how they manage with extremely limited resources. However, it is also important to consider the potential benefits that can be gained from completing an elective within the UK, where you can still step outside your 'comfort zone' and explore opportunities with new client groups, working with other healthcare professionals and in challenging environments.

This chapter will assist you in focusing your ideas for an elective placement and guide you through some of the planning steps while considering the risks and challenges that might lie ahead. It will also help you to identify areas where you may develop personally and professionally and reflect upon learning following the completion of an elective placement.

# Researching the options

Some students may ask the question: Where do I start? There are so many opportunities, both nationally and internationally, that it can be difficult to know where to start looking. Although your university may have some funding available, this should not be taken for granted, so one of the key factors to consider is the budget available. This can then guide your choices from an early stage. If personal commitments and finances are governing your choices, then a UK option may be best. If the budget can stretch further, then an international opportunity may be available to you. Whichever your preference, you need to focus your search and appreciate your limitations. Read Jodie's case study below before attempting Activity 7.1.

---

### Case study: Jodie

Jodie is a second-year adult nursing student who is planning her three-week elective. She has a part-time job and has been saving for a year for this, although she is not sure if she is happy to travel alone but does not know who else to ask. She has asthma and her mother is worried about her travelling abroad. She has always wanted to travel to India. Her other interest is in mental health and she has become interested in the needs of the homeless, particularly those with addictions. The university has links in Brazil and France, but you need to be fluent in the local languages. Jodie has been informed that previous students have used organisations to travel safely abroad, but she is not sure where to start looking.

---

## Activity 7.1   Critical thinking

What key questions does Jodie need to ask herself to facilitate preparation for her elective?

*An outline answer to this activity is given at the end of the chapter.*

As indicated in the above case study, there are many points to consider during the initial stages. Once you have contemplated these, you will be able to start planning your elective and contact potential hosts. It can take months to get a response from some organisations and raising funds can also be time-consuming, so it is never too early to start. Whatever your preference, you will be exposed to a variety of experiences that will give you a broad spectrum for comparisons, whether it is across cultures or just within a new environment.

# Risk assessment/management

Wherever you decide to go on your elective, there will be risks associated with the opportunity. Even if you decide to remain in the UK, you will be attending an area that is unfamiliar to you, with a possibly different group of clients/patients and policies, protocols and procedures. If you are able to travel abroad, there will be a plethora of risks to consider, which may include illness and disease, sanitation, accommodation, cultures and customs, and political issues. Although the potential risks can be minimised by a thorough risk assessment, situations can arise that cannot be predicted, and you will need to be aware of your support network and strategies to limit the impact upon yourself. If you choose to go to a developing country, it is likely that you will encounter much more austere living and working conditions than you have previously been exposed to. While this brings a phenomenal opportunity to experience diverse cultures and differing healthcare provision and practices, you will need to plan carefully. Morgan (2011) has suggested that risks broadly fit into three categories: physical risk to the person, clinical and professional risks, and sociocultural risk. These may not be issues that you have considered, but may include using local transport, being asked to participate in clinical activities that you would not do in your usual practice areas, and language and cultural dress barriers. Morgan (2011) also suggests that students should listen to their inner voice and develop a level of intuitive understanding in order to anticipate difficulties and compare the new unknown with what they are already familiar with.

Your university should provide you with a risk assessment form that will guide you in the areas you need to consider; however, the best place to start is by talking to previous students who have been to the destinations you are interested in and have 'lived the experience'. This can be from previous cohorts or you can browse testimonies that companies publish on their websites. Obviously, you need to read these with caution as they are unlikely to promote themselves with unfavourable feedback. Some countries will be 'out of bounds' due to advice set by the government or because they are not covered by the indemnity insurance you will be required to obtain. As these recommendations can be quite fluid and relate to natural disasters, political unrest and crime rates, it is best to access the government's foreign travel advice website during your planning stages (**www.gov.uk/foreign-travel-advice**) and continue to monitor the relevant web page for your chosen country for any changes that may occur. In general, the RCN, Unison and their counterparts will not provide indemnity insurance for the US or Canada, so unless your university has an arrangement with organisations in these countries, they are usually not suitable for a nursing elective. The following case study might help you to consider issues when risk-assessing an international placement. Then think about the questions raised in Activity 7.2 in relation to Rani's situation.

## Case study: Rani

Rani is considering going to Nigeria for her elective placement but does not know much about the country. She is a child field student but would like to experience care in adult or mental health areas. She is not sure how to find out about suitable areas or what health or cultural risks might be involved. Her interests also include how vaccinations and health promotion are considered in Africa, and she would not like to limit herself to hospital environments. Rani is not sure how to complete her risk assessment form and where to obtain the information.

## Activity 7.2   Decision-making

- Where would you suggest that Rani looks for this information?
- What resources might she have available to her that could guide her decision-making and maintain her safety and health?
- What areas would need to be considered for her risk assessment?
- What support might she be able to expect while she is away?

*An outline answer to this activity is given at the end of the chapter.*

# Further planning points to consider

As highlighted in Activity 7.2, risk assessment is an absolutely essential part of planning the elective journey. Once the risk areas have been given consideration and you have decided where you might wish to go for your elective, you will need to develop your learning objectives and quite possibly write a personal statement to support your application through your university. Some of these points might be quite generalised around learning about new cultures and experiencing healthcare in a new environment, but others will be quite specific to your professional and personal journey so far and relate to what you want to achieve by the end of the experience. Again, you may wish to explore links that your university already has or link this in with the clinical experience you have had so far on your course or in your personal time. Your personal tutor should be able to support you in writing this. You also need to ensure that your visit will be positive for your host and that the experience is not one-sided. Meetoo (2010) discussed a concept known as the 'elective safari', whereby students let their sense of curiosity and spirit of adventure dominate their experience, leading to an inadequate contribution towards the area and a lack of commitment to learning and providing a service. This is not something you would wish to reflect negatively upon you, and it is worth considering your real reasons when making your choices. Nurses can make a valuable contribution to improving health and relieving poverty in low- and middle-income countries given the appropriate tools and support, and you can learn how this is achieved and how you might contribute. Learning objectives for an international elective may include:

- understanding the care needs of children/adults in a different healthcare setting;
- gaining knowledge of the standards of living within a different country and the influences of sanitation and resources on health;
- identifying how privacy and dignity are viewed and maintained in other countries;
- assisting with basic care activities, where appropriate and safe;
- gaining an insight into how individuals with a learning disability or mental health diagnosis are viewed and treated in developing countries;
- appreciating how healthcare is financed in other countries;
- understanding the different training programmes for nursing and how the systems differ from the UK;
- providing healthcare promotion to communities;
- exploring vaccination campaigns and other public health initiatives;
- gaining knowledge around how 'at-risk' groups are managed (e.g. orphans, victims of abuse, the elderly, premature babies);
- comparing how nursing procedures and record-keeping are carried out in another country and the impact of limited resources on quality of care;
- building relationships with staff within other countries to facilitate future work;
- experiencing how children learn to play and the influence of education on their development;
- embracing new environments and developing cultural knowledge;

- understanding the difficulties of living in poverty;
- appreciating how past backgrounds/experiences can have an impact on individuals' daily lives; and
- developing communication skills, particularly across language barriers.

Not all students will be able to travel out of the UK for a range of reasons; it is therefore important to consider what might influence your choice of area and how your learning objectives and personal statement might be developed for a national elective. Activity 7.3 will help you consider this.

## Activity 7.3   Reflection

Although you will have specific placement areas to complete on your course, there are many additional areas you might spend time in that can enhance your learning and professional development. Reflect back over your previous placements and ask yourself the following questions to guide development of your learning objectives and personal statement:

- Is there a client group that I have encountered during my placements that could interest me further, allowing me to experience care in another field?
- Have I had a fantastic outreach experience that I would like to develop into an elective opportunity?
- Is there an aspect of social care that I would like to explore to understand the relationships between health and social care?
- Have I had contact with a charity or specialist organisation during my training so far, and so would like to spend more time with the service?
- Have I had contact with another healthcare professional or a nurse that has inspired me to take a certain direction in my career (e.g. a midwife or paramedic)?
- Would I like to experience nursing in a different part of the country to compare and contrast services and perhaps look for employment opportunities?
- Have I cared for a patient recently where I felt lacking in cultural or social understanding and could not meet their wider physical, emotional, social, economic and spiritual needs? Could I organise an experience that would help me develop this to enhance future care?

*As this activity is based on your own experience, there is no outline answer at the end of the chapter.*

Regardless of whether you are planning to go abroad or stay in the UK, you will meet people from diverse cultures and backgrounds. The next section will help you to consider the skills you have and those you need to acquire in order to develop cultural competence.

# Developing cultural awareness and competence

If you have been reading about the benefits of international placements, you may have come across the term 'cultural competence'. Cultural competence encompasses many different elements and includes the ability to provide care to patients with diverse values, beliefs and behaviours. This will also involve tailoring healthcare delivery to meet patients' social, cultural and linguistic needs, thus addressing any healthcare inequalities. As Norton and Marks-Maran (2014) suggest, to become culturally competent you will need to increase your cultural knowledge, have a sense of personal growth and change your practice, while Standage and Randall (2014) refer to the term 'opening hearts and minds'. They suggest that this will include cultural awareness, cultural knowledge, cultural skill, cultural encounter and cultural desire. None of this will be easy, and you will need to reflect deeply on your experiences to be able to achieve this. Nursing students often express difficulties and challenges meeting the cultural needs of patients. Organising an elective experience, either in the UK or abroad, is one way in which you might be able to address this and enhance your cultural understanding and awareness. To become 'competent', you would first need to develop a cultural understanding or sensitivity. Student nurses who have been on an overseas placement have reported a better understanding of cultural differences and how these may be applied in healthcare (Norton and Marks-Maran, 2014). This may often challenge your existing values and beliefs and require you to 'unlearn' your own cultural values and belief system. You will also need to take time for personal and professional preparation, and when arriving in a new country allow yourself to 'culturally acclimatise'. Duffy et al. (2005) also identify the value of 'transcultural adaptation', which allows students to 'transcend the cultural boundaries', thus experiencing the culture that lies outside the clinical placement. Some students travel early to their elective placement to facilitate this or liaise with their lecturers or organisations to anticipate the dilemmas and frustrations they might encounter. This may relate to something one takes for granted, such as managing without electricity, or as challenging as encountering lack of dignity during end-of-life care or childbirth. You must remember that although this experience will be rewarding, it may be extremely challenging in areas you do not anticipate.

Quappe and Cantatore (2005) suggest that cultural awareness exists at four levels, and there is a concern that when qualified nurses arrive in a new country there is an inherent danger of perceiving that their way of doing things is the only way. Student nurses are generally more aware of their own gaps in knowledge and would not assume that sharing their knowledge and experience is necessarily going to be worthwhile to someone whose cultural background is so different. The four levels of cultural awareness are as follows (you may already be able to recognise where you fit into this relating to your previous experiences within your training so far):

1. My way is the only way. At the first level, people are aware of their way of doing things, and their way is the only way. At this stage, they ignore the impact of cultural differences. (parochial stage)
2. I know their way, but my way is better. At the second level, people are aware of other ways of doing things, but still consider their way as the best one. In this stage, cultural differences are perceived as a source of problems and people tend to ignore them or reduce their significance. (ethnocentric stage)
3. My way and their way. At this level, people are aware of their own way of doing things and others' ways of doing things, and they choose the best way according to the situation. At this stage, people realise that cultural differences can lead both to problems and benefits and are willing to use cultural diversity to create new solutions and alternatives. (synergistic stage)
4. Our way. This fourth and final stage brings people from different cultural backgrounds together for the creation of a culture of shared meanings. People dialogue repeatedly with others and create new meanings and new rules to meet the needs of a particular situation. (participatory third culture stage)

(Quappe and Cantatore, 2005, p2)

There is no suggestion that you need to be at level 4 either before or after an elective placement; this is just to educate you around the findings of previous research and to be aware of your actions and behaviours while you might be participating in an over-seas elective, and to be mindful of the impact your thoughts, feelings and actions might have. Developing cultural sensitivity is an important element of pre-registration pro-grammes within the UK.

You may now question: What would be the benefits of me developing this cul-tural awareness and competence, particularly as it does not seem to be an easy process? Without question, you will need to be flexible and honest, but the ben-efits of immersing yourself within a new culture have been explored. Button et al. (2005) stated that the importance of cultural education within the nursing field has become increasingly important and providing care for patients with culturally diverse backgrounds can enhance the delicate nurse–patient relationship. They also identified that students who participate in transcultural experiences (elec-tives) become more attentive to the subtle difference between cultures and have an increased awareness of local politics and global issues, and that by experiencing differences first-hand they can effectively evaluate the strengths and weaknesses of their own country's healthcare system. Standage and Randall (2014) also supported this throughout their research, whereby student nurses gained a new understand-ing that they could apply to immigrant communities within the UK. While we cannot deny there may be 'uncomfortable situations' that may arise, adequate preparation can reduce the impact of culture shock, and the personal development encountered will outweigh this.

# Experiencing nursing/healthcare in a different environment

While you may be aware that experiencing nursing in a different country can provide students with a broad spectrum for comparison between nursing practices, one must also be mindful that you might be exposed to adverse nursing/healthcare practices that might leave you frustrated. Button et al. (2005) identified that there is literature documenting the impact in disparities in resources, education and even ethics, but students need to be careful about making judgements around another country's healthcare practices. Fundamentally, it will be very challenging to try to change these practices in the short time you are present, and you may need to be aware of how this may affect you, as there is little research around the long-term impact of these experiences. It is vital to reflect on how you might feel when providing care for individuals from different countries and backgrounds. Briscoe (2013) recommended that using a structured critical reflection framework can help create enlightenment especially around emotive concepts, as these may attract strong opinion and are best voiced where there is a climate of trust, respect, openness and safety (Chapter 10 looks at reflection in more detail). The following two case studies describe the experiences for two students during their electives. Read through them and then undertake Activity 7.4..

## Case study: Jack's international elective

Jack is a learning disability field student nurse who went to Jamaica for his placement and worked in a care home that he had organised through family connections. He was really looking forward to his time there, but the challenges were more than he had anticipated. First, he found the heat unbearable and his shifts started at lunchtime, which meant he was in practice during the hottest part of the day. Due to the heat, the odour was also often challenging. He could not stop comparing the nursing practices to that of the UK and was particularly distressed by the lack of facilities that were provided, including no running water. The residents had no privacy, with a lack of curtains and doors, and there was hardly any equipment, particularly for moving and handling, and he said it was really difficult to witness care given in such conditions. He later realised that residents had to pay for mobility aids, and if they could not afford it then they simply went without. Residents who had difficulty in mobility were not given any assistance, and as a result often missed their mealtimes. There was a lack of staff, and residents were often left to help each other; he found that he was often left to help in these situations, which he didn't mind, but he wondered what would have happened if he had not been there. He was really shocked that the

*(Continued)*

(Continued)

residents often had to help with the daily maintenance, such as cleaning, and that security was non-existent. Jack became slightly withdrawn due to his experiences and realised how we take the NHS for granted in the UK. He wondered if he could have acted any differently and if there was anything else he could do on return to the university to complete his final year.

## Case study: Kamandeep's national elective

Kamandeep was a mental health field student nurse who chose to undertake her four-week elective with the paramedic ambulance service out in a rural area where her grandparents lived to make travel arrangements easier. She was considering a career in acute mental health and thought it might give her a different perspective on how treatment would be given during emergencies, including both physical and mental health crises. She went on many 'call-outs' and was exposed to many different clinical emergencies with adults, older people and children. It upset her that the staff she went out with were often judgemental, although they were also reassuring to families, and she found it hard to work out how some patients were taken to hospital against their will while others were left at home when she thought it seemed unsafe. Kamandeep went to a patient with schizophrenia who was disturbed and putting his family at risk, and it was upsetting to see how long they had to wait for specialists. She was also taken to a patient who had taken an overdose; the paramedics declared him 'deceased on arrival', but it distressed her to see they did not attempt to resuscitate him. Kamandeep found the whole pace of the experience very fast and barely caught her breath, although the staff were always checking to see if she was OK. She felt mostly privileged to be part of this care, but in emotional turmoil, and wondered if she was really prepared to be a qualified nurse in a year's time.

## Activity 7.4 Reflection

Reflecting on the two case studies above, how would you have felt if you had been Jack and Kamandeep, and how would you have responded to the events that took place?

- What was Jack's interpretation of the cultural differences he experienced?
- How did he feel towards the residents and staff he met?

- How were his ideals of 'best practice' challenged?
- Could Jack have taken different actions while abroad?
- Could Jack have prepared himself better for his experience?
- How did Kamandeep feel about her colleagues during her placement?
- What were her personal challenges?
- How could Kamandeep have prepared herself in a better way?

*As this activity is based on your own feelings, there is no outline answer at the end of the chapter.*

Looking at Jack's case first, it could be suggested that Jack realised the poor care he witnessed was not due to the lack of professionalism among the staff, but was the 'cultural norm' for this area, and he lacked a sense of cultural competence where he could appreciate the benefits of the cultural differences. Jack possibly felt out of his depth and unable to contextualise his experiences. He had feelings of empathy and compassion for the residents he met and admiration for the staff in their ability to work in adverse conditions; however, he could not understand how they could offer nursing care that did not fit in with his model of best practice. He may have been frustrated that he couldn't make a change. Looking back, Jack may have felt that he should have vocalised his distress at the time and could have made some practical changes. He might have been able to change his shift pattern, and therefore worked in the cooler part of the day. He should have been more prepared for the health systems in Jamaica, and perhaps spoken to other nurses who had visited there and read more about the country and its challenges. He might have had a discussion with the home manager before he left around lack of resources, and even maintained contact after returning home and considered the possibility of fundraising for this area.

Kamandeep, in contrast, was challenged in other areas. She was possibly so busy that she was unable to explore the role of the paramedic at the time the incident with the deceased patient occurred, and possible feelings of helplessness were due to a background in mental health rather than adult health. She may have had a sense of pride in what she was part of and felt admiration for her colleagues, but lacked appreciation of the decision-making and felt confused about the outcomes. Kamandeep was probably not used to a rural environment, where the demands of providing healthcare over a vast area could be different. If faced with this opportunity again, Kamandeep could prepare more fully by researching and speaking to previous students. She could make sense of her emotions by reflecting with her personal tutor to explore in depth why she felt it so challenging and to reassure her that she has not taken the wrong career path.

# Personal and professional development: sharing learning experiences

The way in which you are required to share your learning experience will very much depend on the protocol of your university. Some universities may have the elective linked to one of their modules, which will require a piece of coursework; others may ask you to present a 'conference-style' poster or presentation, or stand up and present to a group of fellow students and/or lecturers. These sessions are usually built into the timetable and occur within a couple of months after you return. Whichever is required, it is important to reflect back over your experience and share the highs and the lows, the challenges and the benefits, and be open and honest with yourself. You may feel that you have matured personally and professionally or that your career pathway has changed and will alter the progression of your postgraduate studies. You might have increased your self-confidence, self-awareness, coping and self-reliance mechanisms or leadership skills. It may be that you now have a greater empathy for a particular group of clients or understanding of a different group of health or social care professionals from outside your field, or you have simply renewed your enthusiasm for your own profession. You may have enhanced your clinical or language skills, become more aware of your non-verbal communication, or overcome personal barriers or previous prejudices. While you were away, you might have made some connections for the next cohort of students or have some tips around how to prepare, minimise risks and get the most out of your electives. It is vital to be creative in sharing your journey, but be mindful of *The Code* (NMC, 2018a) when using photographs and maintaining confidentiality.

## Chapter summary

Looking back over this chapter, we hope that you have a broader understanding of how to research and prepare for an elective placement, as well as how to minimise the risks and accept the challenges. You should appreciate that it is not necessary to travel to faraway places to encounter cultural differences; the challenge of integrating differing beliefs is present in every patient encounter. You should understand that becoming 'culturally competent' is not an easy thing to achieve, but nursing – in any country worldwide – has more similarities than differences. An elective placement, either national or international, requires careful planning, but will greatly improve your nursing knowledge and enhance your professional and personal development. Whichever direction you choose to follow, it is important to reflect on what you have learnt and share your experiences with others in a sensitive manner.

# Activities: brief outline answers

## Activity 7.1   Critical thinking (p123)

Key questions to ask include:

- How will she fund her elective placement, and what is her budget?
- How many weeks does she have for her elective?
- Is there a potential for her to cross fields?
- Does she have any family/friend connections that she could utilise?
- What are her areas of interest, and what sort of placement would she personally gain the most from (e.g. migrant populations, homeless, end of life, global health, social care, acute care)?
- Can she use this opportunity to make links for future career prospects?
- Is she travelling alone or with a colleague/fellow student nurse?
- Can she speak another language?
- Are there any other cultures she wishes to explore?
- Does she have any personal issues to consider before travelling?
- Does her university provide any links with other countries, and where have previous students travelled to?

## Activity 7.2   Decision-making (p124)

First, as there are certain areas that are not safe to travel to within Nigeria, Rani would need to access the Foreign and Commonwealth Office website to refine her search.

To consider health issues and travel advice Rani could also access the website **www.fitfortravel. nhs.uk/home**, which would inform her of immunisations required and other cautions to consider. She could also contact companies that provide trips to Africa for their help and guidance or speak to previous students who have travelled to Nigeria.

Risk categories would include:

- immunisations such as diphtheria, hepatitis A, poliomyelitis, tetanus, yellow fever, hepatitis B, meningococcal meningitis, rabies and typhoid;
- risks of cholera, malaria and Zika virus;
- how to ensure clean drinking water;
- terrorism and crime levels, including political rallies, curfews, and kidnaps and scams;
- safe travel and accommodation;
- rescue and emergency details;
- contingency plans;
- adequate travel insurance, including professional indemnity and possible cover by the university; and
- awareness of local laws and customs, including views of homosexuality, drugs, modest dress, and what you are permitted to photograph (personal safety).

Rani would need to ensure she has supervision from an appropriate individual and remember that throughout her international placement, she is still bound by a professional code, has a duty to act responsibly and ethically at all times, and must not become involved in care where she is unsupervised or for which she has not been trained.

Support available will depend on the university's protocol, but emergency contact information should be provided for insurance purposes. If Rani travels with an organisation, she will have a named link/telephone number to reassure her. Some universities provide face-to-face or online support during the elective using technology; however, many remote areas do not have Internet access.

## Further reading

**Crisp, N.** (2016) *One World Health: An Overview of Global Health.* London: Routledge.

A valuable insight into global health, whether you are travelling abroad or not.

**Lonely Planet** (2019) *The Big Trip*, 4th edn. London: Lonely Planet Publications.

Lots of useful tips if you are travelling abroad.

## Useful websites

Foreign and Commonwealth Office

**www.gov.uk/government/organisations/foreign-commonwealth-office**

A government website that provides global travel advice, including health and safety.

Fir for Travel

**www.fitfortravel.nhs.uk/home**

A public access website provided by the NHS that gives travel health information for people travelling abroad from the UK.

Work the World

**www.worktheworld.co.uk**

An organisation that provides tailored electives in Africa, Asia and Latin America.

Plan My Gap Year

**www.planmygapyear.co.uk**

A volunteer travel organisation, working across 17 countries in Africa, Asia and South America, with opportunities available from 1 to 36 weeks.

Projects Abroad

**www.projects-abroad.co.uk**

An organisation that provides tailored electives in Africa, Asia, Europe, Latin America and the Caribbean.

RCN: Considering an Overseas Elective?

**www.rcn.org.uk/get-help/rcn-advice/student-electives-overseas**

A guide for RCN student members planning an elective placement overseas, including advice on indemnity, finances, visas and travel insurance.

# Chapter 8

# Succeeding in practice when you have additional needs

Robert Stanley

## NMC Standards of Proficiency for Registered Nurses

This chapter will address the following platforms and proficiencies:

**Platform 1: Being an accountable professional**

Registered nurses act in the best interests of people, putting them first and providing nursing care that is person-centred, safe and compassionate. They act professionally at all times and use their knowledge and experience to make evidence-based decisions about care. They communicate effectively, are role models for others, and are accountable for their actions. Registered nurses continually reflect on their practice and keep abreast of new and emerging developments in nursing, health and care.

At the point of registration, the registered nurse will be able to:

1.4 demonstrate an understanding of, and the ability to challenge, discriminatory behaviour.
1.5 understand the demands of professional practice and demonstrate how to recognise signs of vulnerability in themselves or their colleagues and the action required to minimise risks to health.
1.15 demonstrate the numeracy, literacy, digital and technological skills required to meet the needs of people in their care to ensure safe and effective nursing practice.
1.17 take responsibility for continuous self-reflection, seeking and responding to support and feedback to develop their professional knowledge and skills.
1.19 act as an ambassador, upholding the reputation of their profession and promoting public confidence in nursing, health and care services.

**Platform 5: Leading and managing nursing care and working in teams**

Registered nurses provide leadership by acting as a role model for best practice in the delivery of nursing care. They are responsible for managing nursing care and are

*(Continued)*

(Continued)

accountable for the appropriate delegation and supervision of care provided by others in the team including lay carers. They play an active and equal role in the interdisciplinary team, collaborating and communicating effectively with a range of colleagues.

At the point of registration, the registered nurse will be able to:

5.2  understand and apply the principles of human factors, environmental factors and strength-based approaches when working in teams.

**Annexe A: Communication and relationship management skills**

At the point of registration, the registered nurse will be able to safely demonstrate the following skills:

2.9  engage in difficult conversations, including breaking bad news and support people who are feeling emotionally or physically vulnerable or in distress, conveying compassion and sensitivity.

## Chapter aims

After reading this chapter, you will be able to:

- describe what is an additional need, and how it is defined;
- identify who students are with a disability;
- describe what widening participation is and what it means for students with a disability;
- feel more confident to disclose a disability or additional need in practice;
- demonstrate an understanding of reasonable adjustments, what they are and how they can enable you to succeed in practice; and
- identify some of the financial provision available to support students with additional needs.

# Introduction

## Case study: Being a nurse with additional needs – Michelle Quested

Watch the following video on YouTube: **www.youtube.com/watch?v=KmnvQlICzQc**

This is a nurse who is a wheelchair user. Michelle Quested became a wheelchair user following a car accident in 2010 and spent five months in hospital. But she never gave up on her dream of returning to the job she loves, as a neonatal cardiac nurse at Birmingham Children's Hospital, tending premature babies and newborns with serious health problems.

This chapter is about how to succeed on placement if you have additional needs. Michelle Quested is a wonderful example of how an individual can still succeed as a nurse if the right support is in place. Additional needs include dyslexia, a mental health need, dyspraxia, mobility issues, and so on. All universities are legally required to meet those needs to ensure your success on their programmes (Equality Act 2010). However, this chapter focuses on what you, the student, can do if you have an additional need in order to maximise your success in practice. It will define what additional needs are and which fall under the definition of a disability.

This chapter uses a number of video clip examples of students with additional needs within nursing. You are encouraged to use these video clips as a means of gaining a three-dimensional view of a student with additional needs. Indeed, you may have your own story to add.

This chapter is about understanding who the group of students are who have additional needs, what it means for them, what their rights are, and what strategies can be considered to ensure success.

# What is an additional need?

It might be useful to begin by asking the question: What are additional needs? Within the context of this discussion, and considering nursing students in practice, this usually means students with an impairment, activity limitation or participation restriction. 'Disability' is an umbrella term covering all these three elements:

- an impairment is a problem in body function or structure;
- an activity limitation is a difficulty encountered by an individual in executing a task or action; and
- a participation restriction is a problem experienced by an individual in involvement in life situations.

Consider Activity 8.1 to help you understand what these terms mean.

## Activity 8.1 Critical thinking

George uses glasses to enable him to undertake driving, reading, and so on (all activities requiring vision).

*(Continued)*

(Continued)

- Does he have an impairment of body function or structure?
- Does he have an activity limitation?
- Does he have a participation restriction?
- Does he have a disability?
- How would you define disability?

*An outline answer to this activity is given at the end of the chapter.*

Disability is not just a health problem; it is a complex phenomenon, reflecting the interaction between features of a person's body and features of the society in which they live. Overcoming the difficulties faced by people with disabilities requires interventions to remove environmental and social barriers.

The Equality Act 2010 gives a specific legal definition of a person who is disabled:

> *If he or she has a physical or mental impairment and the impairment has a substantial and long-term adverse effect on his or her ability to carry out normal day-to-day activities.*

(S6(1))

This means that, for example, a person with a broken leg or acute infection does not meet the definition, as although they may be very disabled in the short term, this is time-limited and a full recovery can generally be assumed. Equally, a long-term condition that is improved 'by medication, medical treatment or an aid' (Lewis, 2012, p17) may not be classified as a disability because effective management means it does not have an adverse effect on the person's ability to carry out normal day-to-day activities. The range of impairments that might be significant but not create a participation restriction could include physical or sensory impairments such as mobility difficulties, partial-sightedness or deafness, and cognitive impairments or mental health problems such as depression, bipolar disorder or **autistic spectrum disorder (ASD)** (Office for Disability Issues, 2011).

Additionally, there will be students who have additional needs and are adamant they do not have a disability. For some, the word 'disability' carries a stigma:

> *If it says 'are you disabled?' I tend to sort of put 'no, but I have a mobility problem', because I don't class myself as being disabled.*

*Nurse Practitioner*

> *I really don't consider myself disabled, so any sort of question that asks 'have I a disability?' I always say 'no'.*

*Social Work Student*

(Stanley et al., 2007, p61)

Having a disability should not mean someone's contribution is less. People with additional needs bring unique insights and abilities that are invaluable to those they work with and to service users. This is what nursing needs.

In addition, the impact a disability has on an individual and the activities they undertake can vary. For example, impairments that are not generally problematic for the person in their daily life may become problematic for them when training for a nursing qualification. The most common example is that of the wide spectrum of learning difficulties including **dyslexia**, **dyspraxia** and **dyscalculia** (Pollack, 2009). Problems with reading and writing, sequencing, and using numbers that may be managed or avoided in everyday life can become disabling on a nursing programme, as in-depth study, the following of instructions, verbal and written reporting, and drug calculations are critical processes that must be accurate and timely.

These difficulties may not just be struggling to do something, but also struggling with self-esteem. An individual who frequently experiences failure will come to anticipate failure in future endeavours. Failure becomes self-fulfilling as the experience is both reciprocal and reinforcing. Let's look at the case of John to illustrate this and then consider the questions in Activity 8.2.

---

## Case study: John

John is a second-year nursing student who is currently on placement. His grades during Year 1 were poor, with him having to submit a couple of his modules again. Additionally, he is just getting by on placement in terms of learning his clinical essential skills.

On his current placement, John is two weeks into his placement of eight weeks. Already, his practice assessor has concerns and has a meeting with him. She expresses her concerns, in particular that he does not seem to be learning and developing his insight and understanding of the skills required of him, nor performing as expected of a second-year student. She did say he was highly motivated and interested in many things. John said he has always struggled with learning anything, he struggled at school, and had been called stupid many times by many people. He confided to his practice supervisor that he was unsure if he had the ability to be on the course, but he passionately wanted to be a nurse.

The practice supervisor asked what he thought might be affecting his learning, and he said he had recently been diagnosed with **attention deficit hyperactivity disorder (ADHD)**. 'Now it makes sense', said his practice assessor. Understanding his learning needs, she worked out a different process of teaching, and importantly strategies to help him learn the required skills.

He passed his practice placement, and using the same skills passed Years 2 and 3. He is now a staff nurse back at the ward where he previously worked.

## Activity 8.2 Reflection

The practice supervisor's understanding of John's additional learning needs resulted in a positive outcome, but it could have had a very different outcome. Consider the following questions:

1. Why do you think that John was unsure about his ability to be on the course?
2. What would that feel like if you were in the same situation?

*An outline answer to this activity is given at the end of the chapter.*

# Who are the students with a disability?

It is helpful to have an understanding of the population figures with regard to disabilities as many students with (or without) additional needs have no idea how many students on the course have additional needs, and knowing you are not alone can be comforting. Activity 8.3 asks you to consider this.

## Activity 8.3 Reflection

Imagine you are in a lecture theatre with students from your intake. Think about the students in that room:

- How many have a mental health need?
- How many have dyslexia or a specific learning disability?

*An outline answer to this activity is given at the end of the chapter.*

Many students with additional needs think they are the only one, and they are not; they are one of many. In fact, nursing is attractive to many people with a disability often because they have themselves been service users and want to give back to nursing and make a difference. To put the numbers of nursing students with a disability in context, look at Table 8.1, which reports the prevalence of students with declared disabilities on undergraduate nursing programmes in the UK from 2012/13 to 2017/18.

As you can see from Table 8.1, the percentage of nursing students with a declared disability has been rising year on year at an average of 1.21 per cent per year, and has risen by 53.8 per cent between 2012/13 and 2017/2018. Activity 8.4 asks you to consider the implications of these statistics.

| Disability | Academic year | | | | | |
|---|---|---|---|---|---|---|
| | 2012/13 | 2013/14 | 2014/15 | 2015/16 | 2016/17 | 2017/18 |
| A long-standing illness or health condition | 795 | 894 | 992 | 1,090 | 1,237 | 1,398 |
| A physical impairment or mobility issues | 100 | 98 | 118 | 161 | 177 | 191 |
| Another disability, impairment or medical condition | 457 | 486 | 606 | 620 | 682 | 707 |
| Blind or a serious visual impairment | 54 | 45 | 46 | 53 | 67 | 70 |
| Deaf or a serious hearing impairment | 184 | 209 | 223 | 242 | 229 | 229 |
| Mental health condition | 484 | 692 | 915 | 1,169 | 1,544 | 1,975 |
| Social communication/ autistic spectrum disorder | 76 | 79 | 45 | 47 | 58 | 79 |
| Specific learning difficulty | 4,148 | 5,211 | 5,988 | 6,506 | 6,696 | 6,708 |
| Two or more conditions | 204 | 248 | 325 | 459 | 560 | 755 |
| Total | 6,520 | 7,962 | 9,258 | 10,347 | 11,250 | 12,112 |
| No known disability | 52,710 | 57,591 | 60,968 | 63,869 | 66,078 | 65,784 |
| Percentage of nursing students with a declared disability | 12.36% | 13.82% | 15.18% | 16.20% | 17.02% | 18.41% |

*Table 8.1* Nursing students with declared disabilities, 2012/13–2017/18

*Source*: HESA (2019)

## Activity 8.4   Critical thinking

Use Table 8.1 to answer the questions below:

1. What do you think are the implications for nursing of the increasing number of students with a declared disability?
2. Were you surprised by the total of 12,112 students with a known disability for 2017/18? Why? Do you think there are any disabilities (physical or mental) that by their nature should prevent someone from becoming a nurse?

*An outline answer to this activity is given at the end of the chapter.*

Not all students declare their disability when they start their course. Activity 8.5 asks you to consider the implications of this.

## Activity 8.5   Reflection

Many students may not be aware they have an additional need when they first start their nursing programme.

- Why do you think that might be?
- What are the implications of this for their clinical practice?
- What would you suggest should be done to ensure everyone knows all their needs?

*An outline answer to this activity is given at the end of the chapter.*

Widening participation (WP) in higher education has been a major component of government education policy in the UK since the 1990s and will be one of the factors in the increase in students with a disability entering higher education. This policy aims to increase not only the numbers of young people entering higher education, but also the proportion from under-represented groups (e.g. those from lower-income families, people with disabilities, some ethnic minorities). The following video clips offer excellent examples of successful instances of this policy:

- Watch the following video clip on YouTube: **www.youtube.com/watch?v=wV7E_TPy3dc**. In this video, a woman who had grown up with dyslexia tells how the support available gave her the confidence to go to university.
- Watch the following video clip on the *British Deaf News* website: **www.britishdeafnews.co.uk/deaf-dyslexic-nurse-attends-university-20-year-battle/**. This is about Colette Scotton, who has both a hearing impairment and dyslexia, and has fulfilled her ambition after 20 years to study adult nursing at Anglia Ruskin University.

# Declaring a disability

It can be difficult to tell people about yourself and your needs as a student. If you are disabled or have additional needs, you might not want people to know. You may have a condition that no one can see, such as a mental health condition or a specific learning difference like dyslexia.

The following are some things that you might be worried about.

# Will people be less inclined to hire me as a newly qualified nurse if I have additional needs?

No, they won't. Under the Equality Act 2010, prospective employers aren't allowed to ask you any disability-related questions, except to make limited enquiries to ascertain if any reasonable adjustments would need to be made for you. These adjustments could be required at interview or when carrying out the role. They can also ask specific questions to monitor diversity, which are voluntary, so you do not have to answer them if you do not wish. Employers are encouraged to treat disabled candidates more favourably, with the exception of favouring a person with a particular type of disability over another person's impairment.

While on placement, if you demonstrate a professional approach to the management of your disability/long-term health condition while undertaking the programme and you can clearly be seen to have developed as a capable student healthcare professional who also has a disability/long-term health condition, this is likely to be interpreted positively by future employers. References from the university will not divulge any details of disabilities or health conditions.

# Will it affect my ability to do the course?

If you have a disability, health condition or specific learning difficulty such as dyslexia, you may need certain facilities, **assistive technology** or support services to enable you to make the most of your studies and education. This can include alternative examination or assessment arrangements. The Equality Act 2010 calls the arrangements that your university makes to meet these needs 'reasonable adjustments', and they are legally required to do so.

# What should I tell my practice supervisor/assessor on my placement?

Often stigma, or fear of stigma, is one of the main reasons for non-disclosure of a student's disability (Stanley et al., 2007). Students considering disclosure reported their concerns as being perceived or treated as 'different' from their peers:

> *I felt they'd perhaps question my fitness levels or put too much undue emphasis on 'oh she's got a disability, do you know?' and I didn't want to go down that road, I just wanted to be like any other student on the course.*

> (Stanley et al., 2007, p62)

> *It is just that every time she [tutor] sees me she puts her head on one side 'How are you …?' and it is just unbelievable, I think she thinks I am just going to keel over and die there and then and … she treats me like I am like this little special friend who needs to be … I don't know …*

> (Stanley et al., 2007, p66)

143

Both the university and the placement providers understand that you may not wish to disclose personal, sensitive information about yourself; however, it is important that any decision about disclosure is properly informed.

Let's consider some of the advantages of disclosure as seen from a professional perspective. Individual issues can be discussed with the disability coordinators. There are a number of advantages if you disclose your disability in the placement setting:

- Disclosure allows adjustments to be made, which should enable you to fulfil your potential and achieve the learning outcomes of your course.
- When you are working to your potential, then patients/service users/carers will receive better care and staff in practice will be able to support your learning more effectively.
- Disclosure will allow you to concentrate on the work in hand on the placement, free from possible concerns you may have over the concealment of the effects of your disability.
- It is often easier to build an effective working relationship when the people involved feel they can be open about issues that are relevant to the placement. Meeting with the placement staff to discuss your needs can be supported by the disability coordinator or the clinical link if you want to build a relationship with your practice supervisor/assessor before and after disclosing your disability to them.
- You have the opportunity to show how you can perform effectively in the placement setting. For example, you may already have learned many effective ways to communicate and check information that you can explain to your practice supervisor or assessor, forestalling any questions they may have with regard to these activities.
- You may have high levels of empathy with people in your care who have a disability, and in some instances can be a reassuring presence for them.

## How do I tell my practice supervisor/assessor about my additional needs? What should I say? Do I need medical reports?

When you receive your placement allocation, it is recommended you make a pre-visit to discuss your disability and any reasonable adjustments you may have. Managing your disclosure at a time and pace that you choose, and ideally before any issues emerge, enables you to describe your disability in a positive way, as well as any positive effects it has had on your life. For example, if you have a hearing impairment, then your other communication skills may be strong, such as giving attention and use of eye contact or body language. If you have dyslexia, you may have particular strengths in creative thinking and provide innovative solutions to problems. If you want support from the university for this meeting, ask for it. The next case study details Adenrele's experience of seeking support in practice, and is followed by Activity 8.6, which asks you to consider the preparation for practice required for students who have a hearing impairment, as well as how staff and the student involved may feel.

---

### Case study: Adenrele

Adenrele is a student on the undergraduate nursing programme. She has a profound hearing loss and communicates through some lip-reading and the use of sign language interpreters. At the notification of each placement, she goes in advance to discuss her needs and how the practice supervisors and assessor can support her. In many instances, the staff she meets in practice had not worked with a student who used signing interpreters before, and so she found that this meeting before she started was essential so that they understood the role of an interpreter who used sign language and were aware of her needs and could plan for them.

---

### Activity 8.6   Critical thinking

Pre-placement meetings are essential for students with a disability that require one or more reasonable adjustments in practice. Consider the following questions in relation to the case study about Adrenele:

1.   What else do you think should be discussed at the meeting Adenrele has?
2.   What might Adenrele be feeling?
3.   What might the practice supervisor or assessor be feeling?

*An outline answer to this activity is given at the end of the chapter.*

---

# Reasonable adjustments: what are they and what do they mean for me?

The term 'reasonable adjustment' has been used a few times within this chapter to describe the duty to respond to someone with additional needs. The Equality Act 2010 brought together a series of laws that underpin the legal principles of reasonable adjustments. The main laws relating to disability discrimination and to special educational needs in education are:

- Equality Act 2010;
- Disability Discrimination Act 2005;

- Disability Discrimination (Public Authorities) (Statutory Duties) Regulations 2005, SI No. 2966;
- Special Educational Needs and Disability Act 2001;
- Education Act 1996; and
- Disability Discrimination Act 1995.

The Equality Act 2010 imposes a duty to make 'reasonable adjustments' for disabled persons. Reasonable adjustments duty is defined as:

*Where disabled students are placed at a substantial disadvantage by a provision, criterion or practice, the absence of an auxiliary aid or a physical feature, the further or higher education institution must consider whether any reasonable adjustment can be made to overcome that disadvantage.*

(EHRC, 2019)

Disability discrimination in education (as it is elsewhere) is unlawful. Universities must not treat you or any disabled student less favourably than others. They must make 'reasonable adjustments' to ensure that disabled students are not at a substantial disadvantage, and they must prepare accessibility plans to show how they will increase access to education for disabled students over time. Watch the concept of reasonable adjustments summarised in the following video clip: **www.youtube.com/watch?v=pKCP-AxRJTo**

Within practice, the responsibility for those adjustments sits with the placement provider, NHS trust or health organisation. There is a duty to make reasonable adjustments where a disabled student is at a substantial disadvantage. These should be made on an individual basis, involving a process of evaluating what is reasonable within the context of the placement. For example, in the clinical setting, this could include shifting morning shifts if the student is on medication that causes sleepiness.

When deciding if an adjustment is reasonable, factors to be taken into consideration include 'practicality, effectiveness, efficiency, cost, and health and safety (of the individual and others)' (RCN, 2017b, p22). However, there is no duty to make reasonable adjustments that would compromise competence standards; a student with a disability must be able to demonstrate their fitness to practise using reasonable adjustments that do not invalidate competence standards.

For example, in the practice setting, reasonable adjustments for a student with dyslexia may include those that are set out in Table 8.2.

---

**Area of difficulty: memory, listening and speaking**

**On placement, students may have difficulties with:**

- holding on to information for very long;
- remembering when they are under stress, leading to confusion and going into memory overload;

---

- deciding which bits of information are more important than others;

- understanding, following and remembering spoken instructions;

- listening for very long;

- pronouncing words correctly;

- trying to find the correct words to express themselves; and

- sticking to the point when speaking (forgetting the thread).

| Strategies for practice supervisors/assessors: | Strategies for students: |
|---|---|
| • Be patient. | These are some of the adjustments that you, the student, can make within your clinical area in response to dyslexia. |
| • Give verbal instructions in a quiet place if possible. | The importance of this is understanding how the additional need affects you, and then considering strategies in response. |
| • Use straightforward language, speak slowly, pause between phrases and maintain eye contact. | • Practise what you want to say before you meet the person. |
| • Avoid using ambiguous language that could be interpreted in different ways. | • Don't rush when speaking, and pause before answering questions; be brave and say, 'Can I come back to you on that?' if you can't think of what to say. |
| • Give concise instructions in the same order as they are meant to be carried out. | • Stick to the point and speak in short sentences. |
| • Encourage the student to use a notebook to write down verbal instructions; check they got them right. | • Ask the speaker to repeat or rephrase information if necessary. |
| • Be aware of information overload and break down long, complicated instructions into smaller, manageable steps. | • Say the patient's name over and over to yourself; check the client noticeboard and picture their face in your head. |
| • Repeat or rephrase if necessary and emphasise important information. | • 'Anchor' instructions on your fingers. |
| • Say complicated words, medical conditions or drug names clearly, and if necessary ask them to repeat them back to you (suggest they look at **www.howjsay.com** or use a medical dictionary). | • Keep a notebook handy and write down key ideas or words. |
| • 'Anchor' instructions on your fingers (with the student watching) as you say them. | • If you think you're going to forget something, write it down. |
| • Ask the student to repeat back information/instructions while 'anchoring' on their own fingers to ensure they have understood. | • Write down instructions in the correct order.<br>• Ask co-workers not to interrupt. |
| • Provide written instructions if necessary and prioritise tasks/highlight the main points. | • If the speaker is unhelpful (or rude), stress the need for being accurate with information. |
| • Demonstrate practical skills while giving verbal explanations. | • Repeat back information to the speaker to check if it's right. |
| • Encourage the student to audio-record teaching sessions and demonstrations. | • Ask for any practical skills to be demonstrated while listening to verbal explanations. |

*(Continued)*

*Table 8.2*   (Continued)

| | |
|---|---|
| • Encourage the student to repeat back what they have learnt and to reflect on why.<br><br>• Allow the student to practise a task under your observation before meeting the patient.<br><br>• Allow plenty of time during supervisory sessions to explain procedures and routines.<br><br>• Ask staff to avoid interrupting the student while carrying out a task. | • Practise procedures again and again and go through them yet again in your head.<br><br>• Practise saying complicated words or medication out loud; show the word to your practice supervisor and ask how to pronounce it (or use **www.howjsay.com** or a medical dictionary).<br><br>• Build up a glossary of words you use frequently and make sure you can say them.<br><br>• Use the same procedure at handover every time to make it less confusing. |

*Table 8.2*   Adjustments in response to difficulties in memory, listening and speaking

Dyslexia may present challenges in organisation and time management, writing and recording information, and reading. With each of these, there are adjustments the practice area can consider, but importantly adjustments that you, the student, can make for yourself. Different additional needs will have different and individual adjustments. Activity 8.7 asks you to consider the adjustments required for one additional need.

## Activity 8.7   Decision-making

Select an additional need, such as a mental health need, mobility concern or visual impairment. Outline some strategies for succeeding in a practice placement in response to that additional need. Points you may want to consider are:

- Consider any particular worries or difficulties.
- Think about any strategies that you may already have in place to compensate for these difficulties. Think about what skills and strategies you typically use to cope in that situation.
- Can you now think of any other areas of difficulty that you've not yet covered and come up with some possible solutions and strategies?
- Think about how reasonable these solutions and strategies may be in the clinical setting (e.g. audio recording at handover).
- Discuss any alternative strategies that may be more realistic.
- Write down these strategies for further reference.
- Discuss health and safety issues, such as using dangerous equipment and administering drugs, and explore if you may need extra support in these specific procedures.

- Document concerns and strategies.
- Set up regular meetings with the practice supervisor to discuss progress and evaluate how the support strategies are working for everyone.

*As this activity is based on your own choice of an additional need, there is no outline answer at the end of the chapter.*

You should find that your answers in response to Activity 8.7 will all fall under the umbrella of 'reasonable adjustments'.

# Financial help for students with additional needs

Finances are a key consideration for any university student, whether in class or on placement. For many students, going to university is their first experience of paying rent, budgeting for food, and additional living expenses. On placement, there are also the financial demands of transport as an upfront cost, even if this can be claimed back. In 2019, the average expense for just rent and food for an undergraduate student per month was £514 (Save the Student, 2019). This does not account for travel costs, mobile phone, books and social expenses. On top of that, there are tuition fees. UK tuition fees vary depending on your home country.

When on a course, many students undertake part-time employment to provide essential funding, but this may be more problematic for students with additional needs, which is explored in Activity 8.8.

## Activity 8.8 Critical thinking

Students with additional needs may face a number of difficulties in undertaking additional part-time employment. The following questions ask you to consider why, as well as the potential impact on the student:

1. Why might a student with additional needs have fewer opportunities for part-time employment during the course of their studies?
2. How might this affect their additional needs?
3. How might this affect their course of study?

*An outline answer to this activity is given at the end of the chapter.*

On top of the usual loans to cover tuition fees and living expenses, you can get grants towards travel, specialist equipment and non-medical help. If you have an existing care package, this can be transferred to your university. **Disabled Students' Allowances (DSAs)** can be paid in cases of physical or mental impairment, a long-term health or mental health condition, and/or a specific learning difficulty (SpLD) such as dyslexia. Applications for DSAs can be facilitated through the disability services support of the university. It can also be possible for you to get a large room in the halls of residence at the standard room rate, where this is needed as a result of a disability (and not just a physical disability, but also, for example, where a student with ASD will spend much more time than normal in their room). As has been discussed previously, universities are obligated to make your course accessible under the Equality Act 2010, so you can negotiate with them to provide for needs such as specialist equipment, a sign language interpreter, IT equipment, a level access shower, or accommodation for a carer.

Aside from state funding, you can investigate trusts such as:

- Dyslexia Action Learning Fund;
- Gardner's Trust for the Blind;
- Joseph Levy Foundation;
- The Matthew Trust;
- Multiple Sclerosis Society;
- Chrohn's and Colitis UK;
- Snowdon Trust;
- Student Health Association;
- Lawrence Atwell's Charity; and
- The Thomas Wall Trust.

These will give grants for essential study needs that are not covered through other funding streams. Charitable trusts will usually have eligibility criteria that you have to meet in order to get help from them. Getting funds (e.g. grants, student loans, government benefits) for your course can be a lengthy process – UCAS advises that you start applying for financial help six to nine months before a course begins. And of course, the usual rules apply – don't spend it all in the first few weeks of the first term.

# Final reflection

Success in practice with additional needs is about the university, the practice area, and you, the student, understanding those needs and understanding what needs to be in place to demonstrate reasonable adjustments:

> *Inclusive teaching means recognising, accommodating and meeting the learning needs of all your students. It means acknowledging that your students have a range of individual learning needs and are members of diverse communities: a student with a disabling medical condition may also have English as an additional language and be a single parent.*

*Inclusive teaching avoids pigeonholing students into specific groups with predictable and fixed approaches to learning.*

(Open University, 2006)

Disability itself should not be a barrier to nurse education as long as the individual is able to achieve the required competencies, irrespective of impairment or health condition (Maheady, 2006; Marks, 2007).

---

## Chapter summary

A student with an additional need can succeed and become an excellent and valued nurse if the right support is in place. Additional needs can include dyslexia, mental health needs, mobility needs, and hidden long-term health conditions.

Disability is not just a health problem; it is about the interaction between the person and the society within which they live and the barriers that may exist. For the student with additional needs, this will usually mean an impairment, an activity limitation or a participation restriction. 'Disability' is an umbrella term covering all these three elements. The difficulties presented by a disability may be not just struggling to do something, but also struggles with self-esteem.

The number of nursing students with a declared disability has risen by 53.8 per cent between 2012/13 and 2017/18, which is partly due to the widening participation agenda. This has been a major government policy since the 1990s to increase the proportion from under-represented groups (such as people with disabilities) in higher education.

While it can be difficult to tell people about you and your needs as a student with additional needs, there are a number of advantages if you disclose your disability in the placement setting. This will allow the appropriate support to be put in place to support you and enable you to succeed. Disability discrimination is unlawful; universities must not treat disabled students less favourably than others. They must make 'reasonable adjustments' to ensure that disabled students are not at a substantial disadvantage, including practice learning opportunities. Additionally, every student will have developed their own insight and understanding of their additional need, so sharing what helps you can enable practice to provide the adjustments that will enable you to succeed.

---

## Activities: brief outline answers

### Activity 8.1   Critical thinking (pp137–8)

George has an impairment and a participation restriction. He does not have a disability.

## Activity 8.2   Reflection (p140)

It is likely that John lacks confidence, having been told in the past that he is stupid, and so does not believe he can succeed.

Each person will respond differently to a situation such as this, depending on their previous experiences of how people have responded to them. Possible responses are feeling embarrassed, loss of confidence, frustration at not being able to achieve as well as you wish, and anger with yourself or others.

## Activity 8.3   Reflection (p140)

There are many students who have unseen additional needs. Approximately one in six adults has a common mental disorder (CMD) (McManus et al., 2016), and according to the British Dyslexia Association (n.d.) around 10 per cent of the population are affected by dyslexia, so by the law of averages a number of students in your class will have a mental health problem or dyslexia (or both). In addition, a number of students will have long-term conditions that are also invisible, such as diabetes and epilepsy.

## Activity 8.4   Critical thinking (p141)

The implications for nursing are that an increasing non-traditional group of students, some with complex needs, are applying to study. Students with additional needs can bring a lot to the profession as many will be expert patients/experienced service users who can offer a new perspective to colleagues on their experiences.

Depending on your own experience of disability, you may or may not have been surprised by these figures. Applications will be decided on a case-by-case basis in terms of whether the applicant has the ability to meet the NMC proficiencies with reasonable adjustments in place (if required). There should not be a blanket statement that someone with a particular additional need should not be allowed into the nursing profession.

## Activity 8.5   Reflection (p142)

Many additional needs, such as a specific learning difficulty like dyslexia, may be acknowledged during the school years, but not formally diagnosed, or needs may come about as the person grows and life experiences make additional demands on them, as is the case with people with a mental health diagnosis.

The implications for practice are that a student may struggle with certain skills, organising their workload, or managing shift patterns if their disability has not been declared, and so no adjustments have been put in place to support them.

Many universities are now implementing screening processes for a range of needs, such as dyslexia and dyscalculia, to identify students at the beginning of the programme so that support can be put in place early.

## Activity 8.6   Critical thinking (p145)

Things to think about are the impact of the adjustments that Adenrele requires upon the staff and patients/service users in the clinical placement:

- Ensuring patients/service users are informed appropriately.
- Does there need to be adjustment in shifts? Focusing on patient care as well as watching the interpreter can be very tiring, so long days can be difficult for Adenrele, the interpreter and the staff.
- Use of assistive technologies (e.g. recorders) and ensuring confidentiality is not breached.

- Strategies/plans if there is a critical event/crisis in practice and ensuring the safety of Adenrele and the people she is caring for.

Adenrele is likely to be feeling anxious with regard to how staff will respond to her and whether they appreciate what positives she can bring to the placement setting.

Depending on the practice supervisor or assessor's previous experience of supporting a student with a hearing impairment, they may also feel anxious. There may also be concerns regarding the impact of the additional work in supporting a student with a hearing impairment, as well as how patients and other staff may respond to her.

## Activity 8.8 Critical thinking (p149)

Students with additional needs may have fewer employment opportunities. This may be due to issues associated with their physical or mental health impacting on their ability to undertake additional work, in addition to the demands of the course or the challenges with implementing reasonable adjustments. The lack of additional employment, and therefore finance, could adversely impact upon the student's health (e.g. insufficient money to buy balanced meals, pay for heating) and mental well-being (e.g. increased stressors if in financial difficulties). While lack of outside employment should not impact on a student's studies, any negative impact on their physical or mental well-being can have an adverse impact on their studies.

# Further reading

**Hill, S. and Roger, A.** (2016) The experience of disabled and non-disabled students on professional practice placements in the United Kingdom. *Disability and Society*, 31(9): 1205–25.

A study comparing the experience of disabled students in higher education and their non-disabled peers, with an emphasis on practice placements, across six professional disciplines in one UK university.

**L'Ecuyer, K.M.** (2019) Clinical education of nursing students with learning difficulties: an integrative review (part 1). *Nurse Education in Practice*, 34: 173–84.

While American, this is a useful literature review exploring the issues from the perspective of nurse preceptors who educate students and new graduates with learning difficulties in practice.

**Royal College of Nursing (RCN)** (2016) *Reasonable Adjustments: The Peer Support Service Guide for Members Affected by Disability in the Workplace.* Available at: www.rcn.org.uk/professional-development/publications/pub-006595

This guidance is for healthcare professionals with long-term health conditions or chronic impairments.

**Storr, H., Wray, J. and Draper, P.** (2011) Supporting disabled student nurses from registration to qualification: a review of the United Kingdom (UK) literature. *Nurse Education Today*, 31(8): e29–e33.

This paper reviews the UK evidence in relation to support for disabled student nurses from admission to qualification.

# Useful websites

Disabled Students' Allowances (DSAs)

**www.gov.uk/disabled-students-allowances-dsas**

This is the government website for help if you are a student with a learning difficulty, health problem or disability.

Disability Rights UK

**www.disabilityrightsuk.org**

An organisation that enables diverse disabled people to have voice and influence, connecting with each other and themselves.

NOND

**https://nond.org**

An American national organisation for nurses with disabilities. It operates an open membership across disabilities that works to promote equity for people with disabilities and chronic health conditions in nursing through education and advocacy.

RCN: Disability Discrimination and the Equality Act 2010

**www.rcn.org.uk/get-help/rcn-advice/disability-discrimination-and-the-equality-act-2010**

A guide that covers disability and the Equality Act 2010, including who is covered, disclosing disability to your employer, types of discrimination, and challenging discrimination.

# Chapter 9 Raising concerns in practice

Karen Elcock

---

## NMC Standards of Proficiency for Registered Nurses

This chapter will address the following platforms and proficiencies:

**Platform 1: Being an accountable professional**

Registered nurses act in the best interests of people, putting them first and providing nursing care that is person-centred, safe and compassionate. They act professionally at all times and use their knowledge and experience to make evidence-based decisions about care. They communicate effectively, are role models for others, and are accountable for their actions. Registered nurses continually reflect on their practice and keep abreast of new and emerging developments in nursing, health and care.

At the point of registration, the registered nurse will be able to:

1.1 understand and act in accordance with *The Code: Professional Standards of Practice and Behaviour for Nurses, Midwives and Nursing Associates*, and fulfil all registration requirements.

1.3 understand and apply the principles of courage, transparency and the professional duty of candour, recognising and reporting any situations, behaviours or errors that could result in poor care outcomes.

**Platform 6: Improving safety and quality of care**

Registered nurses make a key contribution to the continuous monitoring and quality improvement of care and treatment in order to enhance health outcomes and people's experience of nursing and related care. They assess risks to safety or experience and take appropriate action to manage those, putting the best interests, needs and preferences of people first.

At the point of registration, the registered nurse will be able to:

6.2 understand the relationship between safe staffing levels, appropriate skills mix, safety and quality of care, recognising risks to public protection and quality of care, escalating concerns appropriately.

---

## Chapter aims

..................................................................................................................................................................

After reading this chapter, you will be able to:

- appreciate the importance of raising concerns;
- explain the difference between a concern and a complaint;
- understand the protection afforded through whistleblowing;
- list actions that may constitute neglect or abuse;
- identify the resources available to support you in raising a concern; and
- describe the process for raising a concern.

---

# Introduction

---

## Case study: Owen

..................................................................................................................................................................

Owen was allocated to a GP practice for his first placement. The staff made him very welcome, but when he returned to the university in the second week for a reflection on practice day he asked to talk to his personal tutor as he had some concerns about his placement. He had noticed that when the practice nurse was with patients in the consulting room, staff, including the GP, would simply walk in without knocking to get something from the room or to ask the nurse a question. He felt this was poor practice and showed a lack of respect for the patients' dignity. As it was his first placement, he was unsure what to do and wondered if this was just normal practice and he should just accept that was the way things were in practice.

---

During your programme, you will spend time in a range of different placements and, just like Owen, you will come to each new placement seeing it with fresh eyes. As a student, you will have been shown best practice at university, rehearsing skills in the skills laboratories, and will have been taught about upholding *The Code* and the importance of safeguarding vulnerable people and children. As part of preparation for practice, you will also have been taught about the importance of raising concerns, so it is no surprise that you are likely to be sensitised to the possibility of seeing poor care. As a consequence, you are more likely to pick up on poor practice, as Owen did, than the staff who work there all the time, who may have come to see certain practices as 'normal' or 'acceptable' (Elcock, 2013). While students may pick up on poor practice on their placements, many fear raising concerns about what they see because they believe doing so may have an adverse impact on their assessments in practice or on their experience on future placements in the same organisation. This chapter is designed to help you understand your professional responsibilities with regard to raising a concern and will take you through the process you should follow if you need to raise one. Determining what situations constitute a concern that needs to be raised can sometimes be difficult, so this chapter will explore some of the common types of concerns and discuss the difference between a concern and a complaint. Both universities and health and social care organisations have policies in place, so we will consider the most common ones to help you identify which you need to refer to in different situations. Raising a concern can be quite daunting, so guidance on who and where you can seek support and advice from will be covered, with an explanation on how a concern you raise would be investigated. Finally, the chapter will explain what happens after you have raised a concern.

# Raising concerns as a professional responsibility

*The Code* (NMC, 2018a) describes the standards of conduct and behaviour that are expected of registered nurses, midwives and nursing associates. Although you are a student, *The Code* enables you to understand what it really means to be a registered nurse, and so the professional responsibilities that fall to you. The standards within *The Code* list a number of statements under four themes, and a number of these clearly articulate your responsibility in raising concerns. If you are unsure what your responsibility is, or *The Code*'s directives regarding this, complete Activity 9.1.

## Activity 9.1   Critical thinking

Read *The Code* at: **www.nmc.org.uk/standards/code/**

1.   Which sections of *The Code* provide specific guidance with regard to your role in raising concerns?
2.   Are there any other sections that you think are also relevant to your responsibilities for raising concerns?

*An outline answer to this activity is given at the end of the chapter.*

In fact, if you think about it, failure to comply with any part of *The Code* could put people at risk, and so could be a cause for concern. What is important is the need to recognise that you must always take action whenever you come across situations that put the safety of patients or the public at risk, and in some situations this action cannot wait for you to think about it – an immediate action may be necessary. We will come back to this later in the chapter, but first the next section looks at what happens when people fail to raise concerns, or their concerns are not listened or responded to, in order to help you understand why raising concerns is so important.

# Why the focus on raising concerns?

A number of scandals have been made public regarding failures in healthcare over the last 20 years. These include the death of babies undergoing heart surgery in Bristol (Bristol Royal Infirmary Inquiry, 2001), Harold Shipman, a GP who killed over 200 of his patients (Smith, 2002), the abuse of people with learning disabilities and autism at Winterbourne View Hospital (Flynn, 2012), the death of babies and their mothers at Morecambe Bay Hospital (Kirkup, 2015), and more recently the premature deaths of over 400 people who were given opiate painkillers without reason at Gosport War Memorial Hospital (Gosport Independent Panel, 2018). In each of these cases, concerns were raised by staff and patients/relatives, but their concerns were either not heard or they were not investigated fully. More worryingly was that in most of the above cases, there were healthcare professionals who recognised that there were problems but did not raise any concerns. This is illustrated in great detail in the Francis Independent Inquiry Reports published in 2010 and 2013 (Francis, 2010, 2013). The reports described appalling failures in fundamental care and significant failures at all levels within the Mid Staffordshire NHS Foundation Trust and also externally by key organisations, including Strategic Health Authorities, the NMC, General Medical Council (GMC) and other regulatory bodies, who should have taken action earlier. Accounts from patients and their families described cases where:

- patients were left in excrement in soiled bedclothes for lengthy periods;
- assistance was not provided with feeding for patients who could not eat without help;
- water was left out of reach;
- in spite of persistent requests for help, patients were not assisted in their toileting;
- wards and toilet facilities were left in a filthy condition;
- privacy and dignity, even in death, were denied;
- triage in accident and emergency was undertaken by untrained staff; and
- staff treated patients and those close to them with what appeared to be callous indifference.

(Francis, 2013, p13)

This list covers just some of the findings by Francis in his inquiries. It seems almost incomprehensible that this could occur in a UK hospital, and there are a number of factors that led to these failures. The Francis Independent Inquiry Reports from 2010 and 2013 are very long but are worth reading simply to understand the scale of the failures, what went wrong, and why. Activity 9.2 will help you to explore key areas that Francis reported on.

## Activity 9.2   Critical thinking

The Francis Independent Inquiry Reports, and associated interviews, reports and so on, can be found at: **www.midstaffspublicinquiry.com/report**

Review:

- the executive summary; and
- Chapter 23 in Volume 3, which focuses on nursing.

Looking at the summary of recommendations at the end of Chapter 23, are you aware of any of these that are now in place at your university or on your placements?

*Your answer will depend on your own experiences, but some suggested answers to this activity are given at the end of the chapter.*

The findings in the Francis Reports resulted in a significant shake-up in healthcare regulatory and supervisory systems, and led to a whole series of reviews related to patient safety and roles in healthcare during 2013, including:

- the Keogh Review, which reported on 14 NHS hospital trusts with persistently high mortality rates (Keogh, 2013);
- Don Berwick's report on patient safety within the NHS (Berwick, 2013);
- a review by Neuberger and Aaronovitch of the Liverpool Care Pathway used for people at the end of life (Neuberger and Aaronovitch, 2013); and
- Camilla Cavendish's report on the training and support of healthcare assistants (Cavendish, 2013).

At the same time, the NMC implemented a whole programme of change in response to the Francis Reports, including:

- publication of new standards for pre-registration nurse education in 2010, which included greater emphasis on care and compassion;
- joint development of a guidance document on the professional duty of candour with the GMC in 2015;
- a revised code in 2015 (updated in 2018), with a greater emphasis on the professional responsibility of nurses and midwives to raise concerns and their role in ensuring the fundamentals of care are provided to patients;
- new guidance on raising concerns in 2015;
- the introduction of a new revalidation process for all nurses and midwives, which commenced in 2016; and
- improvements to fitness to practise processes.

What is evident from the above is that the events at Mid Staffordshire had a far-reaching impact, which continues to resonate today. While there are new system checks and processes in place to monitor and assure the quality of health and social care organisations and the registered healthcare professionals within them, these systems are not perfect. Sadly, there are still incidents of poor care being reported at the local and organisational level as new policies and procedures cannot always stop poor behaviour from happening. However, reports and reviews, as well as the creation of new roles and policies, have created greater awareness at all levels. As a consequence, the processes in place to support and enable people to raise concerns have improved significantly, including support for health and social care students. Many of these changes were a direct response to Sir Robert Francis' recommendations for students, universities and placement providers in his report *Freedom to Speak Up: An Independent Review into Creating an Open and Honest Reporting Culture in the NHS* (Francis, 2015). We will look at the support and resources available to you later in this chapter, but first let's look at a common issue raised by students. After reading the scenario, complete Activity 9.3.

## Scenario: Raising a concern

Imagine that you have commenced your placement. Your practice supervisor says she has just had a student and doesn't think it's fair to have another one. Your practice assessor is on annual leave. You are now two weeks into your placement and still have not had a proper induction to the area. You contact the link lecturer to tell them you want to raise a concern about your placement.

## Activity 9.3  Critical thinking

It is likely that you will come across difficult situations similar to the one described in the scenario above, so having a repertoire of possible responses to hand is useful. The following questions will help you to consider how you might respond should anything similar happen to you:

1.  What are your feelings about this scenario?
2.  Why might you have some concerns regarding this placement?
3.  What actions would you take?

*An outline answer to this activity is given at the end of the chapter.*

While the above scenario is concerning, it is not a situation for raising a concern, but it may be one where you would need to raise a complaint. The next section will help you to appreciate the differences between these further.

# The difference between a concern and a complaint

While people are often confused as to whether an issue falls under a raising concerns policy, there is actually a clear difference between a concern and a complaint, and it is important to determine whether the situation you find yourself in falls under a raising concerns policy or a complaints policy in order that you follow the correct process.

The NMC provides the following definitions:

*If you are raising a <u>concern</u>, you are worried generally about an issue, wrongdoing or risk which affects others. You are acting as a witness to what you have observed, or to risks that have been reported to you, and are taking steps to draw attention to a situation which could negatively affect those in your care, staff or the organisation.*

*If you are making a <u>complaint</u> to your employer, you are complaining about how you personally have been treated at work. In these circumstances, you should follow your employer's complaints or grievance procedure.*

(NMC, 2018f, p7)

While the definition of a complaint talks about 'your employer' and 'work', this also applies to you as a student. Where the issue you are raising falls under the definition of a complaint, then you would need to use the placement provider's complaint policy or – if your university has one – a policy or procedure for student complaints within a practice placement setting. It is, however, always better to try to discuss the issues you wish to complain about with those involved first, or with your personal tutor, before resorting to a more formal process. Activity 9.4 is designed to help you consider the differences between concerns and complaints.

## Activity 9.4   Reflection

Think about your experiences in practice so far (or in a previous job or work experience) and reflect on anything that you have seen or been involved in that has concerned you. Can you identify any incidents or issues that you would classify as a cause for concern and any that would fall under the heading of a complaint?

*As this activity is based on your own reflections, there is no outline answer at the end of the chapter.*

Table 9.1 offers some examples that may help you determine whether you have correctly categorised your experiences in Activity 9.4. Once you have looked at Table 9.1, complete Activity 9.5.

| Concerns | Complaints |
|---|---|
| Physical or verbal abuse towards a patient or service user | Verbal abuse by a member of staff against you |
| Evidence of neglect of a patient or service user | Sexual harassment by a member of staff against you |
| Theft from a patient or a ward | Discriminatory behaviour towards you by a member of staff |
| Poor clinical practice | Lack of support on your placement (e.g. no practice supervisor/assessor allocated) |
| A member of staff is physically or mentally unwell but not seeking help | |

*Table 9.1* Examples of concerns and complaints

## Activity 9.5   Reflection

How accurate were you in categorising the issues that have concerned you?

Do you have more examples you could add to the list in Table 9.1?

*As this activity is based on your own observation, there is no outline answer at the end of the chapter.*

Poor clinical practice is the most common concern raised by students and is often related to the failure of staff to follow policies such as failing to wash hands before/ after caring for someone, leaving medications on a locker, or incorrect/unsafe moving and handling procedures.

You may have noted that the first two concerns in Table 9.1 use the terms 'neglect' and 'abuse', and in these cases the concern raised may fall under local safeguarding procedures. 'Abuse' and 'neglect' are overarching terms under which a number of different actions fall, and these can apply to both children and adults. Table 9.2 provides some examples.

| Abuse or neglect in adults | Abuse or neglect in children |
|---|---|
| Physical abuse | Physical abuse |
| Domestic violence | Domestic abuse |
| Sexual abuse/exploitation | Sexual abuse/exploitation |
| Psychological/emotional abuse | Psychological/emotional abuse |
| Financial or material abuse | Female genital mutilation (FGM) |
| Modern slavery | Child trafficking |

| Discriminatory abuse | Bullying/cyberbullying/online abuse |
|---|---|
| Institutional/organisational abuse | Institutional/organisational abuse |
| Neglect and acts of omission | Neglect |
| Self-neglect | |

*Table 9.2*  Examples of abuse and neglect

While you may think that you won't see abuse or neglect on your placements, the Francis Independent Inquiry Reports into the events at the Mid Staffordshire NHS Foundation Trust (Francis 2010, 2013) and the Department of Health serious case review at Winterbourne View (Department of Health, 2012) both detail the abusive conduct of staff in these organisations towards the people in their care. Sadly, neglect and abuse still occur in healthcare organisations, with concerns regarding the treatment of people with learning disabilities in particular constantly in the news (Salman, 2018).

Another factor to take into account is whether what you witness is poor care or a genuine error. Ion et al. (2016) define poor care as involving 'acts of neglect, abuse or incompetence', whereas errors are 'the unintended outcomes of genuine mistakes' (p56). They go on to offer the example of a nurse who makes a drug error and reports it. By following local policy in reporting the error, they would not be deemed to be delivering poor care. However, a nurse who intentionally fails to report a drug error is potentially demonstrating neglect, and so this could also be seen as abuse, in which case this would then be a cause for concern. Obviously, a nurse who repeatedly makes drug errors would be a cause for concern as there is a possible question regarding their competence, and so fitness to practise. Taking these explanations into account, would some of the concerns you identified in Activity 9.5 now fall under errors rather than poor care, and if so are they still a cause for concern?

Another term often linked with raising concerns or making a complaint is 'whistleblowing'. Again, understanding the difference is important, so let's look at this in more detail next.

# Whistleblowing

The terms 'whistleblowing' and 'raising concerns' are often used interchangeably (Ash, 2016). In the UK, whistleblowing describes the act of an employee in raising concerns (which are in the public interest) regarding malpractice or fraud. Employees who 'blow the whistle' are protected under the Public Interest Disclosure Act (PIDA) 1998. Since 2015, the Act has included trainees, which means that you would have the same protection if you made a disclosure as an employee. PIDA protects the whistleblower from harassment or dismissal regardless of whether they disclose internally or to a prescribed person/body, a legal advisor or, if appropriate, a Minister of the Crown. A prescribed person/body is a person or organisation that an employee (or student) can approach outside of the workplace, and we will return to this later.

NHS Improvement (2016) provides the following examples of qualifying disclosures that would fall under the PIDA:

- poor clinical practice or other malpractice that may harm patients;
- concerns about unsafe patient care;
- failure to safeguard patients;
- maladministration of medications;
- untrained staff;
- unsafe working conditions;
- lack of policies;
- a bullying culture; and
- staff who are unwell or stressed and not seeking help.

Unsurprisingly, many of the above are similar to the concerns listed in Table 9.1 earlier. Anyone who makes a disclosure under the PIDA must ensure that it is in the public interest (i.e. the concern you have must affect others and you must be providing information/facts about the concern); it cannot just be an allegation (i.e. without proof).

While all this may seem daunting, the key thing to understand is that you are protected if you raise a concern and have followed the processes set out in the guidance that is available to you. As a student, this means that if you make a disclosure, this should not have a negative impact on your current or future placements or your assessment in practice. There is also a lot of guidance and support available that will help you in raising a concern, so let's explore these resources next.

# Resources available to support you in raising a concern

There are a range of resources available to you that will guide you through the process in raising a concern; which resource you choose to access is likely to depend, in part, on where the concern arises (e.g. placement, work, university) and whether it is actually a concern or a complaint. The main resources will be key people at your university and/or at your placement provider who can guide and support you through the process, along with the local policies available in both organisations. However, there are also a number of websites that provide some easy-to-read advice as well as a range of resources and guidance, including telephone helplines you can call. These resources can be useful to help you decide whether the issue you have is really a concern and needs reporting, and they will also help you to understand what the processes are for raising a concern before approaching anyone formally on the placement or at the university. It is essential, though, that you seek help straight away if someone is at immediate risk or has already come to harm for any reason.

Key people who can help you at your university are:

- your personal tutor;
- the course leader; and
- your academic assessor.

Key people who can help you at your placement are:

- your practice supervisor/assessor;
- the link lecturer;
- the manager in your placement;
- the lead for education at the organisation where you are on placement; and
- the Freedom to Speak Up Guardian (may also be called Champion/Ambassador) based at your NHS/foundation trust.

The Freedom to Speak Up Guardian came into being out of the recommendations by Francis (2015) in his independent review to create a more open and honest culture for raising and reporting concerns in the NHS. Each NHS trust or foundation trust in England now has at least one person in this role; Activity 9.6 will help you to identify who these people are.

## Activity 9.6   Communication

A list of all Freedom to Speak Up Guardians for England is held on the National Guardian Freedom to Speak Up website with their email addresses and phone numbers. Look at the directory of Guardians on their website (**www.nationalguardian.org.uk/**) and look up the NHS trusts you have placements at to see who your local Guardians are.

Make a note of who they are and ask if you can meet with them to discuss their role when you are on placement.

*As this activity is based on your own observation, there is no outline answer at the end of the chapter.*

Were you already aware of Freedom to Speak Up Guardians? Had you been informed of who the Guardians were at your local placement provider as part of your induction? If you were not aware of these roles, feed this back to your university as it can them be included in future sessions on raising concerns.

If you are based in Scotland or Wales, these roles may not yet be in place as they were still being developed at the time of writing. Wales is working on developing NHS

Guardians/Freedom to Speak Guardians and Scotland is developing an Independent National Whistleblowing Officer (INWO). Northern Ireland does not plan, at present, to implement these roles.

If you really felt that you were unable to talk to a local Guardian or felt that your concerns were not being heard, then you could approach one of the prescribed persons or organisations we discussed earlier. This would normally only happen when you had tried raising concerns and felt that your concerns had not been heard, and that the safety of patients or others was at risk. Activity 9.7 will help you identify who the prescribed persons/organisations you can contact are.

## Activity 9.7   Decision-making

Go to the government website (**www.gov.uk**) and search for *Whistleblowing: List of Prescribed People and Bodies.*

1.   What types of people and organisations are listed under 'Healthcare'?
2.   Which organisations are you already aware of?
3.   Which people or organisations would you consider contacting (if any) if you had a concern?

*An outline answer to this activity is given at the end of the chapter.*

Other resources more easily accessible or recognisable that you can access are:

*   the raising concerns policy at the healthcare organisation you are based at –
    NHS trusts in England usually call them a freedom to speak up: raising concerns (whistleblowing) policy;
*   your university's raising concerns policy, which is usually written for all their health and social care students;
*   the NMC's raising concerns website; and
*   the RCN's raising concerns website.

As a student, the most common place for you to come across issues or incidents that are a cause for concern is when you are out on one of your placements. However, issues could also arise outside of placement that would require you to raise a concern. For example, if you have a part-time job or are doing bank or agency work in a health or social care setting, you may come across situations that are a cause for concern. In those situations, you would have to raise the concerns locally using local policies and processes. Another situation you may find yourself in is described in the case study about Senna. Once you have read through the case study, answer the questions in Activity 9.8.

## Case study: Senna

Senna is in her second year. She found her first year challenging as she was a long way from home and struggled with juggling both her academic studies and her placements. You have noticed that she has started to drink quite a lot in the evenings such that she is clearly intoxicated. She has lost a lot of weight and is also looking very pale, with dark circles under her eyes. You have tried to talk to her, and she told you that drinking helps her to relax and to sleep. She said she'd cut down but you have found bottles hidden in the flat. Last night she was doing a night shift and you could smell alcohol on her breath and were concerned that she was not fully sober.

## Activity 9.8   Critical thinking

It can be very difficult when you have a friend who has serious personal problems, but even though you are a student nurse – and not yet registered as a nurse – this is not a situation you can keep secret. Consider the following questions:

1.   Why might Senna's behaviour be a cause for concern?
2.   What actions should you take?

*An outline answer to this activity is given at the end of the chapter.*

It can be difficult to report concerns about a friend or colleague as it may well impact on your friendship with them and could impact on their continuance on the programme or on their job. It can also influence how others may see you. However, these are often the types of reasons given by people who have been involved in the healthcare scandals discussed earlier. As a student on a professional course, you have a professional responsibility to raise concerns that supersedes your relationships with others. This may seem harsh but consider how you would feel if you found out later that because Senna had been drinking, her concentration was poor, and she failed to take the level 2 intermittent observations at the required frequency on a patient who then committed suicide. Earlier identification of Senna's alcohol problem (or her admission that she needed help) would have meant that she could have been referred to services to help her, and her consumption monitored. It would not necessarily have meant that she would be withdrawn from her course.

So, having discussed what concerns are and why it is so important to raise them, let's now look at the process you need to follow to raise a concern.

# The process for raising a concern

The NMC (2018f) describes a number of stages in the process for raising a concern (Figure 9.1). As a student, you would be expected to follow the university raising concerns policy, but it is important for you to understand the NMC's guidance on raising concerns to appreciate the range of options available to you. If you are on an apprenticeship programme or seconded, then you must follow your employer's raising concerns process unless you are on a placement that is outside of your employer's organisation.

Once again, remember that if someone is in immediate harm you should report your concerns immediately to the appropriate person, such as your practice supervisor/assessor, the manager in the placement, or your link lecturer, personal tutor or other member of staff from the university.

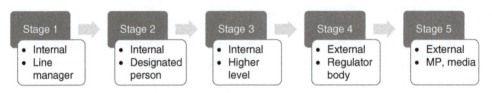

*Figure 9.1*   Stages in raising a concern

*Source*: NMC (2018f)

- *Stage 1*: Talk with the manager in the placement (or someone from the university, if a student).
- *Stage 2*: If you feel unable to talk with the manager, then talk to the designated person within the organisation. This will be detailed in the organisation's raising concerns (whistleblowing) policy (e.g. in England, this would be the Freedom to Speak Up Guardian).
- *Stage 3*: If you feel that your concern has not been managed well, then you can go higher (e.g. the education lead or director of nursing, or even the chief executive).
- *Stage 4*: If you feel unable to raise your concern to anyone within the organisation or you feel that they have not dealt with your concerns properly, you will need to approach someone externally. You can approach a regulatory body. For example, if your concern related to a nurse or several nurses, then you would approach the NMC. If your concern related to the healthcare setting, then you would need to approach the relevant regulator for that organisation. These would include the prescribed persons/organisations discussed earlier and listed in the answer to Activity 9.7 and would include the CQC or Healthcare Improvement Scotland.
- *Stage 5*: If none of the above stages have dealt with your concern appropriately, then you should only consider raising your concern externally with your MP or the media if you have exhausted all other avenues. This is a serious step to take, and advice from your professional body (e.g. the RCN) or trade union is strongly recommended.

Before raising your concern, it is helpful to get your thoughts in order as soon as possible after the incident or incidents you have witnessed. So, writing down what took place in as much detail as you can is important as if it is determined you have a concern that does require investigation then a full statement will be required, and it is surprising how much detail you forget, even over a period of a few days. When you approach someone to raise a concern, they should explain the process for raising a concern with you and the consequences of doing so. You will need to write a statement and make yourself available to be interviewed by the organisation you have raised a concern about, unless you have raised it anonymously.

## Raising a concern anonymously

Students will often ask if they can raise a concern anonymously. The answer is yes. However, if the organisation or person to whom you raise a concern requires more information, they cannot contact you if they do not know who you are. This could limit how far they can proceed with their investigation. Also, it is important to be aware that they cannot feed back the outcome of their investigation to you or any actions they may take as a result of their findings.

# What happens after a concern is raised?

Once you have raised a concern, a discussion will take place with you to understand fully what your concerns are and why you are concerned. If you raised your concerns directly with someone on your placement, then someone from your university should be contacted to support you. You should not go through this process without support from the university, and it is reasonable to ask the organisation to wait to talk with you until that support is available. Following a discussion of your concerns, a decision will be made as to whether your concerns are valid and need to be investigated further. If the decision is made that further investigation is required, it is at this point that you will normally be asked for a formal statement.

Guidance for writing a statement will be provided by your university but can also be found on the RCN website (**www.rcn.org.uk/get-help/rcn-advice/statements**), including the following tips:

- Type double-spaced.
- State who you are and your role (e.g. I am a first-year child field student on a BSc Nursing course from [name of university]).
- State dates and times that any incidents took place.
- Identify who was involved, with their full names and roles/titles, but ensure you keep patients' and relatives' identities anonymous. You can call them Patient A or Patient B, and so on.
- Write your statement in chronological order.

- Ensure you are clear when writing your statement as to what you actually saw, what you may have heard, or what you were told, and by whom.
- Do not use any jargon, and write any abbreviations used in full.
- Describe any actions in detail. For example, if you undertook observations, what time did you do them, and what were they?

(RCN, 2019a)

If you want to raise your concern in confidence, then you must make that clear in your statement or when raising a concern verbally. This means that your name cannot be revealed during the investigation unless there are legal issues raised (e.g. a safeguarding issue involving a child or vulnerable adult, or a criminal offence, in which case your name may need to be revealed to the police or relevant body). You would be informed if this was the case. Your university will support you in writing your statement. At the same time, the university will – in partnership with the placement provider – need to decide whether yourself and any other students on your placement need to be withdrawn from the placement concerned and moved elsewhere. This will be done in discussion with you, and the lead in practice will manage this sensitively. Senior staff in practice recognise that raising concerns is very difficult for students, but as one senior education lead said to me after some students raised a concern in an acute trust, 'These are the nurses we want to employ when they qualify'. You may also be advised to contact your union representative, if you have one, for support and advice.

Once you have written your statement, an investigation will be undertaken by the placement provider. This can take some time and you may be asked to attend a meeting to discuss your concerns further, so ensure that you have kept a copy of your statement that you can refer to. A member of staff from the university will support you at the meeting if you wish or you can ask for your union representative to be present.

The full investigation can take some time depending on what took place and who was involved. You should be kept informed of the progress of the investigation. Once the investigation has been completed by the placement provider, all the key people should be provided with a summary of the key concerns and outcomes and key learning for the organisation and/or university. The key people to be informed will include yourself as the student who raised the concern, placement staff, the senior academic staff member supporting practice or course leader/director, the relevant senior person in practice, and the director of nursing/midwifery.

This chapter has focused on why raising concerns is important and the processes to raise a concern. However, as discussed earlier, it is recognised that it can be very difficult to raise a concern as a student (Francis, 2015). The Council of Deans of Health commissioned a systematic literature review looking at the literature on raising concerns by healthcare students and also included a focus group with students and laypersons (CoDH, 2016). This review and the report by Francis (2015) are summarised in the research summary below.

## Research summary: Raising concerns

The CoDH (2016) systematic review of the literature including a focus group found that healthcare students understood the importance of raising concerns. However, there were concerns about the impact on their relationship with staff on the placement and on their assessment in practice, with some studies reviewed finding students had been failed or marked down in their assessments in practice. Students were also concerned about what might happen if word got out that they had raised concerns and how that might impact on future placements in the same organisation. As a consequence, students either felt unable to raise concerns or would wait until the end of the placement. Francis (2015) found some students disadvantaged if they raised concerns. For example, if they asked to move placement but no placement could be found, they had to make up the time later; in one case, the student was failed as they had not completed their placement.

While this may be concerning, a lot has been put in place since these reports to protect students, including protection under the PIDA and the introduction of Freedom to Speak Up Guardians, as discussed earlier in this chapter, and while some students have had negative experiences, this is not true for all. The key message is that if you have any concerns, talk to someone as soon as possible so that you can get the support needed in raising your concern and writing your statement.

## Chapter summary

This chapter has explored the difficult issue of raising concerns that many students worry about, fearing that it may impact on their continuance on their course. A range of resources have been explored that you can access to support you and enable you to raise a concern using the correct procedures. The difference between raising a concern, raising a complaint and whistleblowing have been explained, as well as the importance of following the correct processes to ensure that you are provided with protection from adverse consequences on your current or future placements. Examples where vulnerable people have suffered abuse or been the recipients of poor care have been discussed to illustrate what happens when concerns are not raised by those responsible for their care or where concerns have not been heard or responded to. Finally, you have been taken through the different stages in raising a concern and provided with guidance on writing a statement, which must be as clear as possible in explaining your concerns to enable a thorough investigation to be undertaken.

# Activities: brief outline answers

## Activity 9.1   Critical thinking (p157)

1.  *Preserve safety* is the key theme focusing on raising concerns. In particular, standard 16 lists six actions and standard 17 lists three actions you must take should there be a risk for patient safety or public protection, or if vulnerable people are at risk. These standards highlight the importance of working within your competence, exercising your professional 'duty of candour', and the need for you to raise concerns immediately if the safety of patients or the public is at risk.

2.  Another section that is also relevant to raising concerns that you may have found is in the introduction to the theme *prioritise people*, which talks about putting people first and making their care and safety your main concern. It provides examples, and standard 3.4 specifically makes clear your role as an advocate for those who are vulnerable and the importance of challenging poor practice and discriminatory attitudes and behaviour. This would also mean raising concerns if no change occurred once you have challenged others.

## Activity 9.2   Critical thinking (p159)

Not all recommendations have been implemented, but possible answers you may have given are:

*   use of values-based interviews at your selection day (e.g. multiple mini-interviews, MMIs);
*   strong focus on compassionate care in your curriculum;
*   revalidation with the NMC now a requirement;
*   ward managers not being counted in the off-duty;
*   a module on leadership in your course; and
*   all healthcare assistants in England and Wales are now required to complete the Care Certificate.

## Activity 9.3   Critical thinking (p160)

1.  Your reactions will probably depend on how many placements you have had and how well they have gone. Delays in the initial interview and induction are not uncommon, and unfortunately not all staff are enthusiastic about having students.

2.  *The Code* clearly states that all staff have a responsibility to support students in practice, and therefore the behaviours of the staff in the scenario are not in line with *The Code*. In addition, induction is an important part of ensuring you are aware of all health and safety considerations in the placement.

3.  Your first point of contact should be the manager in the placement, but if you are not able to do that then contact your link lecturer, who will know the placement and placement staff.

## Activity 9.7   Decision-making (p166)

Key organisations are:

*   professional and regulatory statutory bodies such as the NMC and the GMC;
*   organisations specifically set up with a remit to respond to concerns around quality, such as the CQC; and
*   organisations who have a specific remit (e.g. NHS England deals with matters relating to primary care, medical, dental, ophthalmic and pharmaceutical services in England, and NHS Improvement is responsible for the performance of English NHS trusts).

Specific organisations are provided for Scotland and Wales.

For Northern Ireland, you can go to the following organisations: Regulation and Quality Improvement Authority Northern Ireland, Department of Health, Social Services and Public Safety, and Northern Ireland Social Care Council.

The answers for questions 2 and 3 will be specific to you, but hopefully you guessed the NMC!

## Activity 9.8  Critical thinking (p167)

1. There are two main issues here. It appears that Senna is developing or has an addiction to alcohol, which will impact on her health with potentially serious consequences. In addition, going to work while under the influence of alcohol is a serious concern as she is putting patients and others in her care at risk.

2. If Senna is not responding to your concerns, you should talk to someone at the university; this might be your personal tutor or the course leader.

## Further reading

**Ash, A.** (2016) *Whistleblowing and Ethics in Health and Social Care.* London: Jessica Kingsley Publishers.

A fascinating book that looks at the ethics of whistleblowing, why some people 'blow the whistle' and others don't, and the consequences if they do.

**Fisher, M. and Kiernan, M.** (2019) Student nurses' lived experience of patient safety and raising concerns. *Nurse Education Today,* 77: 1–5.

Provides examples of students' experiences of poor care and how they felt about raising concerns.

**NHS Education for Scotland (NES)** (2018) *Raising Concerns in Practice: Student Guidance – A National Approach for Students, Practice Learning Experience Providers and Higher Education Institutions in Scotland.* Available at: www.nes.scot.nhs.uk/media/4163133/national_raising_concerns_document_with_leaflet_2018.pdf

Useful guidance explaining the process for dealing with instances of poor care witnessed by nursing or midwifery students while on practice in Scotland.

**Nursing and Midwifery Council (NMC)** (2018) *Raising Concerns: Guidance for Nurses, Midwives and Nursing Associates.* Available at: www.nmc.org.uk/globalassets/blocks/media-block/raising-concerns-v2.pdf

The essential guide on raising concerns.

## Useful websites

NHS employers: Raising Concerns (Whistleblowing) – Information for NHS Staff

**www.nhsemployers.org/your-workforce/retain-and-improve/raising-concerns-whistleblowing/information-for-staff**

This web page offers a range of useful resources, including links to useful websites in all four countries of the UK.

Protect

**https://protect-advice.org.uk/**

Formerly called Public Concern at Work, this website provides guidance, support and advice to individuals unsure how to raise a concern, as well as a web page with lots of useful case studies.

Raising Concerns: Guidance for Nurses, Midwives and Nursing Associates

**www.nmc.org.uk/standards/guidance/raising-concerns-guidance-for-nurses-and-midwives/**

NMC website with guidance and a range of useful resources.

Raising Concerns videos

**www.youtube.com/watch?v=a0XWijJ5VuM&t=187s**

**www.youtube.com/watch?v=zjau1Ey0di8**

**www.youtube.com/watch?v=9l5H5UuYufA**

The first video shows Helen Donnelly speaking to the NMC Council about her experience in raising concerns at the Mid Staffordshire NHS Foundation Trust. The second and third videos look at three concerns raised by healthcare staff and how they were followed up on.

Speak Up

**www.speakup.direct/for-employees/**

Provides an online tool to help employees in the NHS or social care settings to decide the best path to take in order to raise a concern. Useful to see different options.

# Chapter 10 Reflecting in and on practice

Kath Sharples and Sonia Levett

---

## NMC Standards of Proficiency for Registered Nurses

This chapter will address the following platforms and proficiencies:

**Platform 5: Leading and managing nursing care and working in teams**

Registered nurses provide leadership by acting as a role model for best practice in the delivery of nursing care. They are responsible for managing nursing care and are accountable for the appropriate delegation and supervision of care provided by others in the team including lay carers. They play an active and equal role in the interdisciplinary team, collaborating and communicating effectively with a range of colleagues.

At the point of registration, the registered nurse will be able to:

5.7  demonstrate the ability to monitor and evaluate the quality of care delivered by others in the team and lay carers.

5.8  support and supervise students in the delivery of nursing care, promoting reflection and providing constructive feedback, and evaluating and documenting their performance.

5.9  demonstrate the ability to challenge and provide constructive feedback about care delivered by others in the team, and support them to identify and agree individual learning needs.

5.10 contribute to supervision and team reflection activities to promote improvements in practice and services.

---

## Chapter aims

After reading this chapter, you will be able to:

*   appreciate the value of reflective practice;

*(Continued)*

(Continued)

- identify a range of reflective models to inform your practice;
- select from a range of reflective models to support differing practice situations; and
- appreciate the role of reflective practice in evaluating nursing care and promoting improvements in practice and services.

# Introduction

There is an expectation that all nurses will reflect on practice, either as part of their day-to-day role, to support learning within a course of study, or to inform revalidation. Reflection is therefore an essential skill for you to develop, as it will form a vital aspect of all future nursing practice. This chapter will provide an overview of reflection and explore some of the more popular reflective models you can use. The models will be discussed in relation to differing types of practice scenarios, exploring how you might choose the most appropriate reflective model from the range available. Discussion of reflective models in relation to positive experiences as well as challenging situations will aid understanding of the links between reflection and the ability to lead nursing care and work in teams. Practical applications, such as the value of keeping a reflective journal to support revalidation, will also be addressed. Lastly, this chapter will enable you to identify how reflection can be used to identify future learning needs to enhance future placement experiences.

# Learning to reflect

As you begin this chapter on reflection, it is important to note that the concept of reflection is not unique to nursing, as it is one of the many ways that we make sense of our life experiences (R. Middleton, 2017). No matter your age or personal circumstances, your life experiences prior to commencing your nursing programme will have exposed you to situations where reflection could easily have been incorporated into your daily routine. However, reflection should never be confused with just looking back on situations or events; thinking about an experience is not the same as reflecting on an experience. Without a structure, just thinking about a situation can result in rumination rather than reflection. Learning how to reflect is an essential skill for you as a student as it enables you to learn from experience, it is often used as a basis for assignments, and it is an NMC requirement of all registered nurses. If these skills are not developed, you are putting yourself at risk of ruminating about your practice rather than reflecting.

# Reflection or rumination?

Reflection and rumination are very different to each other, although on the surface they can appear very similar as they do share some common features. To eliminate confusion, it is important that we begin by defining exactly what we mean by rumination as opposed to reflection so we can tell them apart (Figure 10.1).

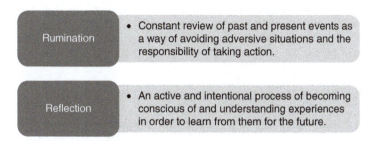

*Figure 10.1*  Definition of rumination and reflection

*Source*: Lengelle et al. (2016)

Based on these definitions, it is possible to begin identifying some of the key differences between rumination and reflection in relation to nursing practice. Whereas reflection involves a thinking process that leads to insight (Asselin et al., 2013), by contrast rumination involves a bottomless pit of thinking, characterised by loss of spontaneity and even pessimism (Van Woerkom, 2010). It is clear that reflection involves far more than just thinking about a situation; rather, it provides nurses with strategy for responding to complex, changing situations in order to minimise risk and develop competence (Lengelle et al., 2016). Reflection is not just looking back; it is looking back in order to process experiences with the intention of moving forward (Morris, 2014).

# The value of reflection

When used correctly, reflection can provide a powerful means of not just seeing previous experience from a new perspective, but as a way of developing critical thinking and crucial insight (Asselin et al., 2013). When used incorrectly, reflection can result in little more than introspection, which many student nurses describe as navel-gazing (R. Middleton, 2017). If nurses do not develop these skills, they may be at risk of developing anxiety and depression due to excessive rumination. Repeatedly ruminating on practice experiences without a reflective framework can cause feelings of inadequacy; in turn, this can raise anxiety and interfere with the ability to solve problems (Werenberg, 2016). For example, Taylor et al. (2015) report that nurse managers must buffer the enormity of their work challenges with reflective processes to reduce the potential for feeling drained and depleted. However, one aspect of reflection that is often overlooked is its value in identifying what you have done well, and so helping you build your confidence in your practice.

Reflection is such a fundamental aspect of improving practice that it is found throughout pre-registration nursing curricula. It is likely that you have been required to reflect individually and in groups as part of self-directed learning, tutorials, online activities and assessments (R. Middleton, 2017). It is likely you feel that you are being asked to reflect all the time! You will find that there are many different reflective models available, although your university may suggest you use one specific module on your course. In this chapter, we will explore three of these models. Before we do that, complete Activity 10.1, as the work you do for this will be used throughout the chapter.

## Activity 10.1   Reflection

The activities throughout this chapter are designed to help you to identify appropriate reflective models to apply to differing practice situations. To get the most out of these activities, it is best if you pause here and take the time to select an experience from practice or simulation that you would like to explore further through reflection. Ideally, the practice experience should be a situation where you were directly involved rather than just observing others. Try to select a situation where you can easily recall what you were doing, thinking and feeling before the event took place, while the event was happening, and the thoughts and feelings you may have experienced after the event. While there is no right or wrong practice situation that you might select, it is helpful if you select a practice situation where you may have encountered some personal or professional challenges as this will add to the richness of your learning. If the situation resulted in what you now recognise as rumination, this is an ideal opportunity to identify how reflection would have helped you to work through the experience differently.

As you will be asked to return to this practice experience throughout the chapter, take some time to choose an experience that you would like to revisit on multiple occasions as you build your knowledge and understanding.

Pause now and write out a brief description of the experience so you can refer back to it as you move through the chapter.

*As this activity is based on your own observation, there is no outline answer at the end of the chapter.*

# Reflective models

There is a vast array of reflective models that are suggested as frameworks for reflection, so an exhaustive explanation of all reflective models is outside the scope of this chapter. Instead, the focus of this chapter will be on exploring just three of the more popular models that can be used by students and registered nurses for reflection in and on practice. If you would like to explore additional reflective models, a number of suggestions are made for further reading at the end of the chapter.

## Johns' reflective model

One of the more common reflective models used in nursing practice is commonly referred to as 'Johns' 10th'. He has constantly refined his model, so much so that there are many versions of it available; in fact, his latest version is number 17. The origins of Johns' model can be traced back to Carper's fundamental ways of knowing in nursing, described in Table 10.1 (Carper, 1978). Johns (1995) acknowledges that the great achievement of Carper was to challenge the tendency of defining, and thereby limiting, nursing knowledge exclusively to empirical measures. Carper recognised that in addition to empirical insight, the dimensions of aesthetic, personal and ethical ways of knowing are required in order for nurses to embrace, know and value nursing care and knowledge. Without this insight, nurses may be limited to viewing their practice as a series of rules and processes that they need to perform with the primary goal of getting the job done (Sumner, 2010). Not only does this promote inflexible and concrete thinking; it also tends to relegate patients to the status of depersonalised objects that need to be crossed off a list according to a strict timeline (Sumner, 2010). Johns (1995) built on Carper's original work in two main ways. First, he outlined a series of 'cue questions' for each of Carper's categories that would assist nurses to frame their learning through practice. He also identified that nursing knowledge requires an understanding of what Carper (1978) defined as interrelatedness. For this reason, Johns' reflective model includes an additional theme of reflexivity with associated cue questions (Figure 10.2). This may sound a little confusing, as Johns uses words you may not be familiar with, but hopefully it will become clearer by completing Activity 10.2.

| Empirical knowing | Knowledge that comes from research, observation and objective facts |
|---|---|
| Personal knowing | Knowledge of ourselves – comes through observation and reflection, the therapeutic use of self in developing authentic personal relationships |
| Ethical knowing | Knowledge of what is morally right and wrong |
| Aesthetic knowing | The art of nursing, the ability to emphasise and understand the individual's experience |

*Table 10.1*   Carper's fundamental ways of knowing

*Source:* Carper (1978)

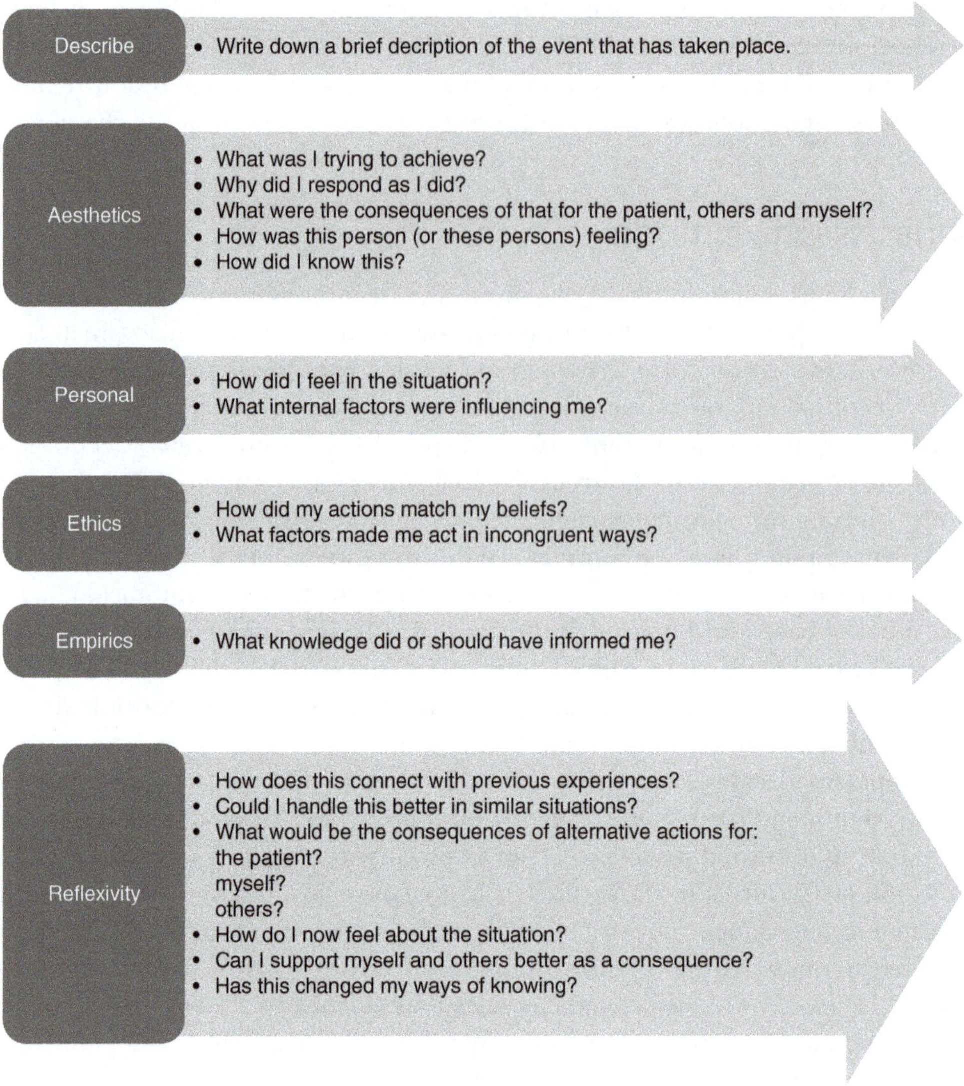

| Describe | • Write down a brief decription of the event that has taken place. |

| Aesthetics | • What was I trying to achieve?<br>• Why did I respond as I did?<br>• What were the consequences of that for the patient, others and myself?<br>• How was this person (or these persons) feeling?<br>• How did I know this? |

| Personal | • How did I feel in the situation?<br>• What internal factors were influencing me? |

| Ethics | • How did my actions match my beliefs?<br>• What factors made me act in incongruent ways? |

| Empirics | • What knowledge did or should have informed me? |

| Reflexivity | • How does this connect with previous experiences?<br>• Could I handle this better in similar situations?<br>• What would be the consequences of alternative actions for:<br>the patient?<br>myself?<br>others?<br>• How do I now feel about the situation?<br>• Can I support myself and others better as a consequence?<br>• Has this changed my ways of knowing? |

*Figure 10.2* A model of structured reflection

*Source*: Adapted from Johns (1995)

## Activity 10.2   Reflection

Refer back to the practice experience you described in Activity 10.1. Use the categories and cue questions depicted in Figure 10.2 to reflect on your experience using Johns' reflective model. Take note of how your understanding may change as you work through the model.

*As this activity is based on your own observation, there is no outline answer at the end of the chapter.*

# Gibbs' reflective cycle

It is highly likely you have heard of Gibbs' reflective cycle (Gibbs, 1988). Deriving its origins from Dewey's model of reflective learning (Dewey, 1933), Gibbs' reflective cycle is very popular for use in nursing programmes, and is just as likely to be familiar to student nurses in Australia as it is to student nurses in the UK (Figure 10.3). In order to appreciate its simplicity, complete Activity 10.3.

| Cycle stages | Reflective cues |
|---|---|
| Description | What happened? |
| Feelings | What were you thinking or feeling? |
| Evaluation | What was good/bad about the situation? |
| Analysis | What sense can you make of the situation? |
| Conclusion | What else could you have done? |
| Action plan | If the situation arose again, what would you do? |

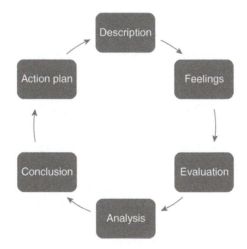

*Figure 10.3*   Gibbs' reflective cycle

*Source:* Gibbs (1988)

## Activity 10.3   Reflection

Refer back to the practice experience you described in Activity 10.1.
Use the categories and cue questions depicted in Figure 10.3 to reflect
on your experience using Gibbs' reflective cycle. Take note of how your
understanding may change as you work through the model.

*As this activity is based on your own observation, there is no outline answer at the end
of the chapter.*

The popularity of Gibbs' reflective cycle is no doubt due to the fact that it is transferable across both theory and practice and is relatively easy to remember (Sharples and Elcock, 2011). Whereas Johns' reflective model is intended to guide a written piece of work, Gibbs' reflective cycle can be used to guide either reflective writing or reflective discussion. As a student nurse, you may find that you are first introduced to Gibbs' reflective cycle in the theory part of your curriculum, where the cue questions assist you to structure a reflective essay or portfolio entry. The fact that Gibbs' reflective cycle is used by many universities as a way to structure a written reflection about a practice experience can reinforce the myth among nursing students that it can only be used for written reflections. However, the six stages of the model can also be used for guiding a formal reflective discussion or informal debrief about a practice experience (Sharples and Elcock, 2011). An example of how this might be achieved is provided in Petra's case study.

## Case study: Petra

I remember being on a placement in an older adult mental health unit in my third year. One of the service users was morbidly obese and we used a standing hoist every day to help him move from the bed to the chair. He became very unwell one day and we needed to get him back into bed quickly. There were lots of nurses around and everyone started struggling with how to get him out of the chair. It was a bit of a disaster, to be honest. I tried to speak up and suggest a different type of hoist that I'd seen in the storeroom, but it was hard because everyone was speaking at once. I went to get the hoist and then found the storeroom locked, and it took me ages to find the keys. Eventually, I returned with the hoist, and when the other nurses saw what I was doing we all worked together to get him back into bed. We had a debrief about it after; I was praised for my quick thinking and was commended for my contribution in keeping everyone safe. We didn't call it a structured reflection, but I realised later that we had actually gone through Gibbs' reflective cycle that we'd been taught at university. We all talked about how we had felt, what was good and bad about the event, and how difficult it was when we were not listening to each other. Everyone was keen to talk about what we could have done differently and lots of people came up with suggestions. We decided to find a different place on the unit to store the hoists so they weren't in a locked room, and moved them to the new location the same day. It was great teamwork.

## Rolfe's reflective model

In recent years, Rolfe's reflective model (Rolfe et al., 2001) has gained increasing popularity within undergraduate and postgraduate nursing curricula. Rolfe's reflective model expands on three questions devised by Borton (1970) – 'What?', 'So what?' and 'Now what?' – by adding additional questions that are generic, easily adapted to suit most nursing situations, and form a reflexive cycle (Rolfe et al., 2001). It can therefore be easily used in both formal and informal reflective opportunities, and can support both written reflections, reflective discussions and reflection during practice (Figure 10.4). Activity 10.4 is the last of the activities asking you to apply your original reflection from Activity 10.1, this time using Rolfe's reflective model. Hopefully, you are now getting the feel for reflective writing.

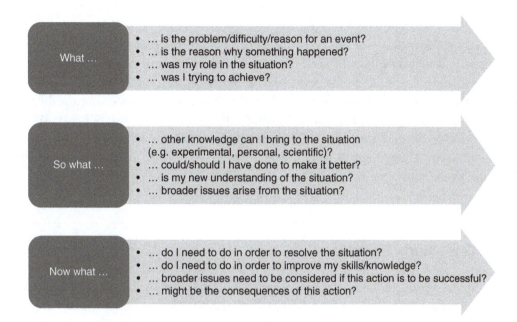

*Figure 10.4*   Rolfe's reflective model

*Source:* Adapted from Rolfe et al. (2001)

## Activity 10.4   Reflection

Refer back to the practice experience you described in Activity 10.1. Use the categories and cue questions depicted in Figure 10.4 to reflect on your experience using Rolfe's reflective model. Take note of how your understanding may change as you work through the model.

*As this activity is based on your own observation, there is no outline answer at the end of the chapter.*

# Reflecting in action

The term 'reflection *in* action' is used to identify the ability to reflect on what is happening while it is happening and adjust as needed (Schon, 1983). If you have already undertaken a placement, then you will have had opportunities to reflect in action. For the majority of students, their first experience of reflection in action happens unconsciously and will have started immediately upon entering the practice area. Likewise, if you have experienced practice via simulation activities in skills labs, you will also have been exposed to reflecting in action, although you may not have been aware of it at the time.

It is common for students to undertake a practice placement without being aware of the opportunities for using reflection in action to enrich their learning. You are probably very familiar with the little voice inside your head providing constant rapid-fire feedback on what you are encountering but haven't realised that this internal dialogue is the early stages of reflection in action. The reason for this is related to the way this internal dialogue is processed. If the reflection is too superficial, this will generally do little more than reinforce thoughts, as opposed to opening up the possibility for new thoughts and considering alternative solutions (Fowler, 2014). Without a framework, you may find yourself entering into a downward spiral of rumination rather than an upward spiral of learning through reflection in action, as shown in Grannie's case study.

## Case study: Grannie

About a year ago, I did a practice placement in a children's ward. I was asked to complete the pre-op checklist for Raheeb, a 7-year-old boy who was returning to theatre for reversal of his colostomy. The ward where I was placed was using electronic records. I forgot to use my login to do the checklist as it was already logged in as the nurse I was working with. When I realised that I'd documented under another name, I didn't say anything. I didn't want to cause trouble and I didn't want the ward manager to know I'd made a mistake. In the end, I just thought no one would find out. When we got down to theatre, the checklist was reviewed by the nurse in the transfer bay and it all came out. I had to own up and say what I'd done. The nurse in the transfer bay was annoyed and kept repeating that she shouldn't really accept the patient, and did I know how serious this was. Raheeb started to cry; he thought something had gone wrong, and the next thing he was screaming at his mum. All these people rushed in to see what all the yelling was about. The more people that came, the more distressed Raheeb got. That's when Raheeb's mum refused to let him go into theatre. She said she didn't trust the hospital any more, that if they got a checklist wrong then they might do the wrong operation. There was no way to change her mind. She had withdrawn consent and Raheeb went back to the ward without having the operation. It was all my fault. I went to the bathroom and just burst into tears. It was awful; I had two days left on my placement and I called in sick both days. I kept thinking about what had happened for weeks. I remember not sleeping well and I'd get this really shaky feeling from time to time. All this happened almost a year ago and I still feel sick when I think about what happened. I never did find out what happened to Raheeb.

In order to prevent internal feedback descending into rumination, a reflective model needs to be incorporated into the experience while it is happening. It is this process that allows for adjustments to be made while the experience is taking place; as a student nurse, you can then use reflection in action to transfer your practice experiences into learning opportunities (Sharples, 2011).

Grannie's experience in the case study is a prime example of rumination rather than reflection. She could have used reflection in action to think through the implications of using someone else's login details to document the care given in the patient's electronic record. If she had reflected in action, she would have been able to think through the consequences of not saying anything versus telling someone of her error. This would have resulted in a relatively straightforward solution. Without a reflective framework, however, Grannie was unable to identify the likely consequences of her error, and a correctable documentation mistake turned into a cancelled operation and a distressed child and mother. Activity 10.5 will help you to reflect on the different models we have introduced in this chapter.

## Activity 10.5    Critical thinking

Based on the reflective models we have covered so far in this chapter, which framework do you think Grannie could have used in this situation to support the need for reflection in action?

*An outline answer to this activity is given at the end of the chapter.*

As reflection is often synonymous with attributes of critical thinking (Price, 2004), reflection in action is far more than just raising awareness of experiences; it is the process that is used to make sense of and learn from the experience while it is happening. Mastering reflection in action will not only play a key role in determining how you feel during your placement, but also what and how much you are able to learn.

# Reflecting on action

Reflection *on* action refers to the reflective thinking that takes place after an experience in a post hoc manner (Schon, 1983). Reflection on action can cause considerable discomfort as it exposes nurses to thinking about themselves in relation to the whole patient care episode rather than just focusing on individual nursing tasks that are either done or not done, as shown in Susan's case study. Activity 10.6 asks you to consider the best model for Susan to use.

## Case study: Susan

When I was in my third year, I had my final placement in PACU. I was working with Ravi, one of the experienced nurses, and we accepted an unconscious patient with a laryngeal mask airway from theatre. I successfully removed the airway and then Ravi said I was capable of managing all of the post-op assessments and observations by myself. I remember feeling so proud of myself. After about 20 minutes, another patient came out of theatre, and as my first patient was stable Ravi asked me to look after them as well. The second patient was in a lot of pain and needed analgesia. I asked for Ravi to help me make up the medication and administer the boluses, which he did. It took about 40 minutes for the patient to feel more comfortable. Then Ravi asked me why my first patient was still in PACU. He said they had been in PACU for over an hour and I needed to get them back to the ward so I could take another patient. I couldn't believe it. Ravi knew I was busy with my second patient administering pain relief; of all people, he should have known why it was impossible to discharge the patient when my other patient was in so much pain. I was seething; why could he not understand that there was nothing I could do? I went from feeling great to feeling terrible. I didn't talk to him for the rest of the shift and I asked not to work with him again.

## Activity 10.6   Critical thinking

Based on the reflective models we have covered so far in this chapter, which framework do you think Susan could have used in this situation to support the need for reflection on action?

*An outline answer to this activity is given at the end of the chapter.*

# Learning through reflection

Many students find that their focus during practice placements is on completing tasks (Sumner, 2010), with the aim of getting 'signed off' on their proficiencies. Focusing on developing nursing skills to the point where they have become automatic is sometimes referred to as low-road transfer (Salomon and Perkins, 1989). While low-road transfer may appear as if learning is taking place, it generally results in nursing care being performed without mindfulness or careful deliberation (Sung, 2006). If you continually adopt a low-road transfer approach during your practice placement, you will no doubt participate in many tasks and eventually find that you learn some things via repetition (Sharples, 2011). You may even find that you can appear to be developing competence by formulaic copying of skills (Sung, 2006). However, with little understanding of the significance of the tasks and skills you are performing, the mask of competence will eventually slip. As an experienced nurse once said, 'You need to be careful not to think that confidence equals competence'.

In order to demonstrate the knowledge, skill and professionalism required for competence, you will need to develop a high-road transfer approach to learning. High-road transfer prompts questions, comprehension and self-regulation (Sung, 2006). Rather than being preoccupied with duties and tasks (Sumner, 2010), high-road transfer paves the way for alternative approaches and viewing nursing care beyond illness and treatment options (Benner, 1984). By using both reflection in action and reflection on action, you can open the gate to high-road learning, and so develop a tolerance for the uncertainty, ambivalence and ambiguity you will encounter in healthcare (Avis and Freshwater, 2006).

With such a variety of reflective frameworks from which to choose, you may find it difficult to translate these theoretical reflective frameworks into your day-to-day practice. You are not alone. A study on reflection in practice found that while most experienced nurses spontaneously reflected, they rarely used a formal framework, and while they found reflection useful for gaining insights, they did not systematically implement practice changes as a result of reflection (Asselin et al., 2013).

# Maintaining a reflective journal

Engaging with a reflective journal is one way to learn how to translate your practice experiences by using a reflective framework. Grasping the fundamentals of reflection in action and reflection on action will not only provide rich opportunities to learn; a reflective attitude will support you in developing competence. As we have already discovered, if reflection is absent from the practice experience, learning is quickly stunted. It is reflection that allows nurses to stand outside of the patient experience and think objectively (Sumner, 2010).

Maintaining a reflective journal does not have to be time-consuming, and as you gain experience your journaling will become quicker and easier (Sharples and Elcock, 2011). Maintaining a reflective journal can be valuable if you don't know where to begin and is especially useful in learning how to structure a reflection on action. In fact, many students find that once they have started to use a reflective journal, they are better able to perform reflection in action, as the case study about Sunni shows.

## Case study: Sunni

About three years ago, I was on my last placement as a student and allocated to a busy haematology ward. Lots of the patients were prescribed IV antibiotics.

*(Continued)*

(Continued)

The medication rounds were always extra busy as most of the time the antibiotics came in powder form; they had to be reconstituted with sterile water first and then made up into 10 ml of sodium chloride before being administered as an IV bolus. Sometimes, if the nurses were really busy, I noticed that the total volume of the IV antibiotics would be a bit more than 10 ml. As the patients always received the full amount in the syringe, I didn't think it really mattered. I wrote about this in the reflective journal I was keeping for the placement because I was still trying to decide if having more than 10 ml was a medication error. I remember using Rolfe's reflective model to structure my reflection, and when I got to the 'So what?' section I realised that this was an example of a medication error. If the antibiotic was over-diluted, it might have been the right dose but not the right volume. I used 'Now what?' to confirm that the total volume of all IV medications must be exactly as prescribed in the BNF. Just last week, I was making up an IV antibiotic for a patient and realised that the total volume was 11 ml. I automatically just went to the sink, discarded the dose and started again. There was a third-year student in the treatment room at the time, and she saw what I was doing and asked why. I explained myself using the 'What?', 'So what?' and 'Now what?' framework. It suddenly dawned on me that I had just turned a reflection on action journal entry that I hadn't thought about for three years into a personal reflection in action, and then translated this back to a reflection on action as I passed on my knowledge to the student.

You can see from the case study that reflection is not just something to use as a student and then forget about once you are a registered nurse. The reflective skills you learn while you are a student will not only aid your learning on practice placement, but also provide the insight you need as you progress through you career. It is very common for newly qualified registered nurses to first realise the value of practice reflection as they adjust to their recently acquired accountability and responsibility (Sharples and Elcock, 2011) and need to use it for their NMC revalidation following their initial registration.

# Reflecting to learn

Remember that the purpose of reflection is not to look back and ruminate; it is to move forward and grow. Reflection can assist you to make sense of particular situations or events and appreciate what you know and have learnt. It can also help you to set learning objectives or goals for areas for further development. Activity 10.7 provides you with the opportunity to practise setting learning goals that you can use for future placements.

## Activity 10.7 Critical thinking

At the beginning of this chapter, you were asked to document a practice experience that you would like to explore further through reflection. This activity will demonstrate how it is possible to use reflection to develop future learning objectives.

Start by choosing a whole placement or simulation that you would like to reflect on. Use Rolfe's reflective model to review your experience, focusing on the overall learning experience rather than just a singular event. As you work through the process, try to stay focused on how you can use what you have learnt from this experience in future placements. You could use the template below to make some notes.

| Reflective stages | My reflection |
|---|---|
| What? | |
| So what? | |
| Now what? | |

*An outline answer to this activity is given at the end of the chapter.*

# Revalidation and reflection

Revalidation refers to the process that all NMC registrants must undertake in order to maintain their registration with the NMC (2019). Revalidation is a continuous process that you will need to engage with throughout your career, and you will be required to participate in revalidation to maintain your registration. Reflection is included within the revalidation process and will form part of the evidence you provide to the NMC to demonstrate your continued ability to practise safely and effectively.

You will see from Figure 10.5 that written reflections are required as part of the evidence all nurses must supply for revalidation. The NMC sets requirements for what can be included in reflective accounts (e.g. continuing professional development, practice-related feedback or practice experiences). As each nurse must supply evidence of five written reflections as part of the revalidation process, it is recommended that reflective accounts are written throughout the registration period, and not left to the 60 days before your registration is due.

**Evidence required for revalidation**

√ 450 practice hours for each registration (dual registration – e.g. nurse and midwife – requires 900 practice hours)

√ 35 hours of continuing professional development (of which 20 must be participatory)

√ Five pieces of practice-related feedback

√ Five written reflective accounts

√ Health and character declaration

√ Professional indemnity arrangement

√ Confirmation

*Figure 10.5*   Checklist of requirements

*Source*: NMC (2019)

# Reflective account

The NMC requires nurses to submit their five reflective accounts on the form that is available to download on the NMC website and shown in Figure 10.6.

| **What was the nature of the CPD activity and/or practice-related feedback and/or event or experience in your practice?** |
|---|
| |
| **What did you learn from the CPD activity and/or feedback and/or event or experience in your practice?** |
| |
| **How did you change or improve your practice as a result?** |
| |
| **How is this relevant to *The Code*?** <br> Select one or more themes: prioritise people – practise effectively – preserve safety – promote professionalism and trust |
| |

*Figure 10.6*   Reflective accounts form

*Source*: NMC (2019)

In addition to reflective accounts, the NMC also requires nurses to provide evidence of a reflective discussion with another NMC registrant as part of the revalidation process. The topic of your reflective discussion must be based on your five written reflective accounts and must also be completed on the form provided by the NMC.

Given the importance of reflection in order to learn from practice, develop competence and provide evidence for revalidation, many students begin documenting their reflective journal as part of their learning during practice placement and then continue to develop this over time into a professional portfolio. As e-portfolios are also available for storing evidence (Reed, 2015), it is relatively straightforward to document a detailed record of your nursing career. Not only can a portfolio include a reflective journal to support your practice learning as you advance through your degree; it can also be developed into a record of your placement experiences by adapting the NMC CPD log, a place to maintain all of your professional documents and a rich source of information to include in your professional CV. Creating and maintaining a professional portfolio also enables you to identify your strengths to develop a plan to address any learning needs (Cope and Murray, 2018). If you would like to commence an e-portfolio, we recommend that you do some background research and find one that suits your needs as a student but is also flexible enough to grow and develop with your career. A good starting point is to ensure that the e-portfolio is compatible with the mandatory forms required by the NMC and does not have limitations to the storage capacity.

## Chapter summary

This chapter has explored what it means to reflect on practice, either as part of a practice placement or via simulation. Learning the skill of reflection as a student is a vital aspect of all future nursing practice. Three of the more popular reflective models have been discussed throughout the chapter in relation to some practice case studies, exploring how you might use reflection to learn, develop competence and work in teams. More practical applications, such as the value of keeping a reflective journal to support revalidation and development of a professional portfolio, have also been addressed. In reading this chapter, you should now have a clear understanding of how reflection can be used to identify future learning needs to enhance future placement experiences.

## Activities: brief outline answers

### Activity 10.5   Critical thinking (p185)

Rolfe's reflective model would have been a good one to use to reflect in action. At the time Grannie realised what she had done with the documentation mistake, she could have used the 'So what?' process to identify that the mistake would be picked up when the checklist was reviewed in theatre. Grannie would have known that this would cause a delay. Realising this, Grannie would have realised that 'Now what?' she needed to do was speak to another nurse and correct the error before Raheeb went to theatre.

## Activity 10.6   Critical thinking (p186)

If Susan had used a reflective model that supported reflection on action, she would have been able to understand the situation better and develop her own knowledge and skills in the PACU environment. Either Gibbs' reflective cycle, Rolfe's reflective model or Johns' reflective model could have been used. Whichever model Susan felt most comfortable with would have allowed her to question why other PACU nurses could care for more than one patient at a time. She could have identified that Ravi was unlikely to have given her responsibility beyond what she could reasonably handle, especially as he had always been supportive on every other occasion. Reflection would have allowed Susan to ask other nurses about their strategies for time management and developing skills for prioritising care in a busy and fast-paced environment. She could have planned ahead to decide how she would alter her practice if she were to encounter the same situation in the future. She may even have identified that Ravi would be a great person to speak with about this; his years of PACU experience meant that he frequently cared for multiple patients and he always appeared so calm and in control. In fact, reflection would have perhaps encouraged Susan to think of Ravi as the best nurse to learn from rather than the nurse she had decided to avoid.

## Activity 10.7   Critical thinking (p189)

| Reflective stages | My reflection |
|---|---|
| What? | During my assessed medication administration simulation in the lab, I was failed because I forgot to do hand hygiene. I thought this was really unfair as I got everything else right and I'm still annoyed that they picked up on something so small. |
| So what? | So what if I forgot hand hygiene? It's a simulation and not a real patient. Mind you, I guess the whole point of simulation is to perform exactly what needs to be done in practice. So, what would be the consequences if I forgot hand hygiene with a real patient? When we looked at the research on hospital-acquired infections last year, there was so much evidence about C. diff being spread due to ineffective hand hygiene. We even had a case study about patient deaths on a care of the elderly ward because of a C. diff outbreak. |
| Now what? | In less than one year, I'm going to be a registered nurse. It won't be a simulation anymore; I'll be caring for patients with no one to check I'm doing hand hygiene. If I forget, I could really harm someone; I could be the cause of a patient getting a hospital-acquired infection. What will I do then? It will be so much worse than just having to redo a simulation. The reason I didn't do hand hygiene in the simulation was not because I don't think it's important; it's because I was so focused on doing the medication administration that I forgot everything else. If I forget something when I'm a registered nurse, someone could die. I'm going back to the simulation lab to ask for a practice session so that I can get this right. |

# Further reading

**Esterhuizen, P. and Howatson-Jones, L.** (2019) *Reflective Practice in Nursing*, 4th edn. London: SAGE.

Aimed at students; a great guide to help you develop your skills in reflection.

**Johns, C.** (1995) Framing learning through reflection within Carper's fundamental ways of knowing in nursing. *Journal of Advanced Nursing*, 22(2): 226–34.

Explains how Johns' model for reflection was developed.

**Schon, D.** (1983) *The Reflective Practitioner*. San Francisco, CA: Jossey-Bass.

The seminal text that explores and explains the process of reflection used by professionals.

# Useful websites

NMC Revalidation

**http://revalidation.nmc.org.uk**

The NMC have provided this website as a step-by-step guide through the process.

Reflective Practice

**www.youtube.com/watch?v=r1aYWbLj0U8**

In this YouTube video, Dr Phillip Dawson from Monash University provides an overview of reflective practice and also addresses some of the anxieties some might experience about the process.

# Chapter 11 Preparing for employment

Jane Dundas

## Chapter aims

After reading this chapter, you will be able to:

- recognise the legal and regulatory requirements that govern your learning in practice during your transition to become a registered nurse;
- identify the key skills and abilities essential for employment during your transition to become a registered nurse;
- describe some of the qualities and skills required for effective leadership;
- identify areas for personal development of your own leadership qualities and abilities during your transition to become a fully qualified nurse;
- demonstrate understanding of the value of preceptorship in development of your leadership skills; and
- identify strategies to choose your first post and prepare for that crucial first interview.

# Introduction

No matter whether you are at the start of your course or nearing the end of your time in university, you may have mixed emotions about what lies ahead. You will feel excited at the prospect of becoming a registered nurse, but you may also be feeling anxious about the future. These are emotions experienced by many university students, but research has shown that nursing students are subject to increased psychological pressures, especially during the period of transition to registered nurse at the end of your studies (Doody et al., 2012). There is no doubt that nursing offers a wonderful career choice full of opportunities, but as you progress through the course you will become increasingly aware of your professional responsibilities for providing safe and effective care. In order to prepare you for some of the challenges that lie ahead, this chapter encourages you to explore some of the ways in which you can develop your own personal qualities to enable you to work effectively in a team. We will also consider some of the key areas seen as important by employers (e.g. delegation, accountability and development of leadership skills). You may not think of yourself as a leader and you may believe that this is an unrealistic expectation at this early stage of your career, but there are many practical ways to overcome your reservations, and this chapter will set out some simple steps to support and guide you to identify your learning needs. We will also explore some of the themes that nursing students commonly identify as beyond their comfort zone, such as overcoming conflict situations and assertive communication, and look at strategies for developing these skills through your placement experiences. The chapter also offers some guidance to enable you to make the best choice for your first post and to prepare yourself for that all-important interview, as well as considering the value of preceptorship.

We will start off by looking at delegation, which is one of the most common sources of students' anxiety and is also one of the skills essential to acquire before you qualify.

# Delegation
## What is delegation?

*Delegation is defined as the transfer to a competent individual, of the authority to perform a specific task in a specified situation.*

(NMC, 2018g, p3)

What does this mean in practice? If you're delegating a task, it's your responsibility to make sure that:

- delegation does not harm the interests of people in your care;
- the task is within the other person's scope of competence;
- the person you are delegating to understands the boundaries of their own competence;
- the person you are delegating to understands the task;
- the person you are delegating to is clear about the circumstances in which they must refer back to you;
- you take reasonable steps to identify any risks and whether any supervision might be necessary; and
- you take reasonable steps to monitor the outcome of the delegated task.

(NMC, 2018g, p4)

For further guidance to improve your delegation skills, read the NMC's supplementary information to *The Code* (NMC, 2018g).

## Delegation and effective teamwork

Delegation is a useful management tool, which when used effectively will enhance your abilities as a leader as you progress in your career. As a student nurse, you should aim to practise and perfect your delegation skills; this will enable you to manage your workload and prioritise tasks and responsibilities to make more effective use of your time. Delegation can help to build relationships and trust with your team colleagues; it can also be an empowering development strategy for junior colleagues when done in a supportive way. As you progress through the course, notice how it feels when someone delegates a task to you, particularly if they delegate well. For example, do you feel encouraged and supported? Do they check that you understood the task? Do they ask what you have learnt from doing the task?

When you qualify and it is your turn to delegate, remembering these experiences will enable you to become a role model for other students learning to delegate.

# What is your delegation style?

It is important to consider your own delegation style in the light of recent research, which suggests that newly qualified nurses adopt a range of delegation styles, summarised in Table 11.1.

| Delegation style | Descriptor |
|---|---|
| The do-it-all nurse | Completes most of the work themself |
| The justifier | Over-explains reasons for decisions and is sometimes defensive |
| The buddy | Wants to be everybody's friend and avoids assuming authority |
| The role model | Hopes that healthcare assistants will copy their best practice but has no way of ensuring how this is done |
| The inspector | Is acutely aware of their accountability and constantly checks the work of healthcare assistants |

*Table 11.1* Delegation styles

*Source*: Magnusson et al. (2017, p48)

If you recognise yourself as following one of these styles, it is a good idea to read the complete article, which will help you to understand some of the factors that lead student nurses (and you) to behave in this way. The researchers found that the most commonly used style was the 'do-it-all nurse', which was largely due to a lack of confidence. Nurses said that they did not want to tell healthcare assistants (HCAs) what to do because they believed that HCAs were more experienced. The researchers observed that this belief resulted in poor teamwork, with poor communication and a lack of interaction between HCAs and nurses, even though they were working alongside one another.

The following case study is an example of the consequences of one student's attempt to delegate; the student has given her permission to share her story.

## Case study: Delegation challenges

On the third week of placement, my mentor assigned me to manage a bay of four patients working with a healthcare assistant (HCA), Sonya. I had access to my mentor, who was on the same shift, but she was working across the whole ward so not directly supervising my practice. I started taking and recording patients' observations while Sonya made beds. I had to take handover for an emergency admission to the bay, which meant that I had to stop doing observations in order to prioritise the new patient's care. I delegated the remaining observations to Sonya while I completed the admission paperwork for the new patient. Sonya told me that she was busy with

*(Continued)*

(Continued)

bed-making and refused to help with the vital observations. Sonya was an experienced HCA and older than me, and I thought she might have felt offended that a student could tell her what to do. I decided I needed to be firm and repeated my request for her to complete the observations, which she reluctantly did. Once I had made the new patient comfortable, I went over the observation charts to ensure they had been appropriately completed, but this upset Sonya and she became angry and told me I did not trust her or believe she knew what she was doing.

Consider the student nurse's behaviour in the case study above to help you complete Activity 11.1.

## Activity 11.1   Team working

Using Table 11.1, consider the following questions:

1.  What delegation style or styles did the student use?
2.  What else could the student have done to make sure that team working with Sonya went more smoothly?

*An outline answer to this activity is given at the end of the chapter.*

# Fear of delegating

The fear factor can also impact on your ability to delegate well; these are some of the common fears that student nurses express:

*   Fear of criticism: *Will I lose respect?*
*   Fear of liability: *Will I be blamed for the mistakes of others?*
*   Fear of loss of control: *Will the job be done right?*
*   Fear of overburdening others: *They are already too busy.*

If you ever find yourself feeling like this, you need to face your fears and adopt the development strategies below when you are next in placement.

The following are suggested strategies to help you improve your delegation skills:

*   Practice delegation – set yourself a target to delegate to someone at least three times a week.
*   Ask your colleagues for feedback about your delegation style, in particular the person you delegate to.

- Be honest if you lack confidence – discuss ways to improve your confidence levels with your practice supervisors.
- Read up about delegation and familiarise yourself with the key principles.
- Observe other nurses who delegate well and use their example to model your behaviour.
- Identify your learning and development needs as part of your reflection (see Activity 11.2).

However, it is important to remember what delegation is *not*:

- It is *not* just a way to offload work.
- It is *not* giving and following orders.
- It is *not* just doing what you're told.

Accountability is another area that worries students, and it is important to realise that when you delegate you are accountable for your actions. The following section and activities will help to clear any doubt.

# Accountability

The NMC defines accountability as follows:

> *Accountability is the principle that individuals and organisations are responsible for their actions and may be required to explain them to others.*

(NMC, 2018g, p3)

This means that you accept full responsibility for your actions and you are able to provide a satisfactory reason for your decision to act. You may think that as a student nurse, this does not apply to you, but the law imposes a duty of care on all practitioners, whether they are a student, a healthcare assistant or a registered professional. Your understanding of accountability will become increasingly relevant as you progress through the course, when you will be encouraged to become less reliant on the supervision of qualified staff and begin to work more autonomously and take more initiative. Always remember that as you become more independent and confident in your practice, you are still required to work within the limitations of your level of competence; it is when you accept responsibility for a task that you then become accountable. To consolidate your learning so far, undertake Activity 11.2.

## Activity 11.2   Leadership and management

Watch the RCN online resource on accountability and delegation (**www.rcn. org.uk/professional-development/accountability-and-delegation**), which outlines some of the principles of accountability and patient safety in relation

*(Continued)*

(Continued)

to delegation. Note down any changes in your understanding of your role in leadership and management and keep for Activity 11.3.

*As this activity is based on your own observation, there is no outline answer at the end of the chapter.*

Taking time to think about your experiences and what you have learnt is important. Reflective writing is a skill that some students find challenging to do well at first, but reflection is an essential part of your development as a nurse and reflecting on your experiences will also help you to develop resilience and become a lifelong learner. If you have not already done so, read and complete the reflective activities in Chapter 10 in preparation for Activity 11.3, which requires you to reflect on your practice and write two short pieces about your experiences of delegation.

## Activity 11.3   Reflection

Write a short reflective account about your experiences of delegation in practice:

1. where someone delegated a task to you; and
2. where you delegated a task to someone else.

Apply the principles of accountability and delegation and ask yourself the following questions:

1. Was the delegation carried out effectively in each case?
2. What evidence do you have to support your answer?
3. If the delegation was not effective, what could be done differently in the future?
4. How does your ability to delegate effectively inform your leadership development?

Then note down some key actions for the future development of your delegation skills.

*As this activity is based on your own observation, there is no outline answer at the end of the chapter.*

Now that we have covered some key skills for leadership, let's look at leadership itself in more detail.

# Leadership and management in nursing

If you have been a student representative or team captain, or have organised an event or played a leading role in other ways, you may already feel confident in your abilities to lead and influence other people; however, many student nurses will not yet have acquired these skills. Leadership is nothing to be intimidated by; it is a skill like any other and can be learnt and developed in practice. Activity 11.4 will get you started.

## Activity 11.4   Leadership and management

Taylor and Fontaine (2019) have some useful activities you can undertake to help you develop your leadership skills. In addition, see the following videos and use them to help you identify some strategies to enhance your leadership/management skills when you are next working in practice:

Molly Case: Nursing the Nation
**www.youtube.com/watch?v=XOCda6OiYpg**
Professor Michael West: Leadership in Today's NHS
**www.youtube.com/watch?v=0RXthT32vcY**
Michael West: Collaborative and Compassionate Leadership
**www.kingsfund.org.uk/audio-video/michael-west-collaborative-compassionate-leadership**

*As this activity is based on your own observation, there is no outline answer at the end of the chapter.*

When you think of leadership in nursing, think of it as an opportunity to provide the best care for patients and to ensure their safety. The first step towards development of your leadership abilities is to develop self-awareness; becoming aware of your own responses and behaviour will enable you to empathise with your colleagues and become more influential.

# Developing self-awareness

Health Education England (HEE) developed a model of leadership development for undergraduate nurses based on evidence from a national research project. You can use this model, described in the research summary below, as a focus for your own leadership development throughout the course of your studies.

---

## Research summary: Leadership model

The three stages of developing as a leader during pre-registration education are identified as:

- *Stage 1: Focus on self.* Developing self-awareness and self-efficacy to foster understanding of one's own beliefs, attitudes, values, knowledge, attributes and skills in order to build and develop leadership behaviours.
- *Stage 2: Working with others.* Understanding how one interacts and connects with the diversity of other people in organisations and learning how to develop positive team working in a multi-professional and complex clinical environment.
- *Stage 3: Improving healthcare.* Developing and leading teams to instigate and action positive change in practice to assure quality, safety of care and continuous improvement of services through evidence-based approaches.

(HEE, 2018)

---

There are many tools and techniques that will help you to understand your own cultural values, preferences, beliefs, attitudes, strengths and limitations, which will help inform development of your leadership behaviours and abilities. Developing your sense of self and understanding who you are will enable you to develop your professional identity and will determine how you lead. There are links to various self-assessment resources suggested at the end of this chapter; exploring these resources will afford you opportunities to reflect on your behaviour, but you may benefit from discussing and comparing your findings with your fellow students. You can also seek constructive feedback from your peers to see if they agree with any new insights you have gained. Feedback from others is the best way to identify aspects of your behaviour that you may be unaware of.

When you completed the reflective exercises earlier in this chapter and in Chapter 10, you will hopefully have understood that reflective practice is key to developing self-awareness; it is also instrumental in developing resilience and self-efficacy. Being aware of your own emotional responses to challenging situations in practice is a fundamental part of learning to manage and cope with the unexpected (Jackson et al., 2011). As HEE (2018) state:

> *Ultimately, it is critical that the student explores themselves and harmonises their identity as a professional, a leader and as a unique individual and feels at ease with this.*

(p18)

As you begin to become more self-aware, you will learn to recognise the aspects of others' behaviour that might make you become emotional or angry; sometimes this can happen quite suddenly and lead to a conflict situation. Conflict is part of normal life in a busy organisation, and many student nurses are unsure what to do. The next section offers some strategies to prevent and cope with conflict situations.

# Coping with conflict

Your colleagues, relatives and patients may also experience intense, angry reactions as a result of working under pressure or being confined in a highly charged, stressful environment such as a busy ward. One of the strategies that will enable you to cope with any conflict situation is to avoid taking it personally. Conflict can be a positive force for change and improvements in practice, but when handled badly it can be destructive (Jones and Bennett, 2012, p91). NHS Improvement (2018) has produced an excellent guide to managing conflict, which is especially useful when conflicts arise as a result of uncertainty and change. The guide highlights three main sources of conflict (Table 11.2).

| Form of conflict | Descriptor |
|---|---|
| 1. Task conflict | Includes differences of opinion, viewpoints and ideas. Some task conflict can actually be beneficial to the change process as it enables people to discuss a more diverse range of views and ideas before making decisions. |
| 2. Process conflict | Involves disagreement over the logistics of achieving an outcome or change (e.g. who takes on which responsibilities or who delegates to whom). |
| 3. Relationship conflict | Often the most destructive form of conflict and takes the form of perceived interpersonal incompatibility between people. This may be on the basis of personal values, morals or personality characteristics. |

*Table 11.2* Forms of conflict

*Source:* NHS Improvement (2018)

Understanding the root cause of a conflict situation will enable you to work out a mutually agreeable solution. Keep your cool and try to calm tempers, give people the benefit of the doubt, and understand that people may just be having a bad day outside the workplace. Relatives or patients may have a justified reason for being upset, but it is worthwhile considering your colleagues' responses with a similar degree of kindness and patience. Maintaining an attitude of positive regard for others is a code of behaviour that will help you to gain mutual respect and enable you to become an authentic leader. Keep in mind the principles of conflict resolution, summarised in Figure 11.1.

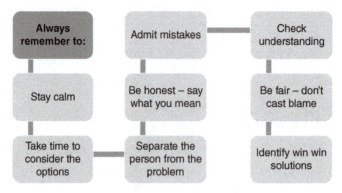

*Figure 11.1*   Principles of conflict resolution

Another strategy to help you cope with conflict is to be aware of your natural style, based on your assertiveness and cooperativeness. The five conflict management styles are shown in Figure 11.2, which provides information useful for completing Activity 11.5.

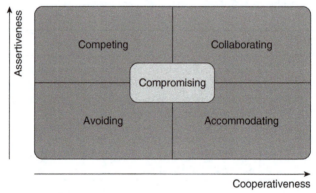

*Figure 11.2*   Conflict resolution styles

*Source*: Thomas and Kilmann (1974)

## Activity 11.5   Communication

This activity will help you explore your conflict management style and apply it to a recent conflict situation (see also Figures 11.1 and 11.2).

1.   Complete the conflict self-assessment questionnaire listed in the useful websites at the end of this chapter.
2.   Reflect on a recent conflict situation you were involved with:

  •   What was the nature of the conflict?
  •   What style did the other person adopt?

- What conflict style did you use?
- On reflection, what do you notice about the conflict now?
- What could you have done differently?

*As this activity is based on your own observation, there is no outline answer at the end of the chapter.*

## Trigger points

In order to empathise with the responses of other people, it is worthwhile reflecting on your own trigger points. Have you ever experienced a sudden emotional or angry response to a particular situation, seemingly out of the blue? For example, someone points out that you have not done something well, or perhaps you think they are being overly critical about your work. You might not have consciously realised, but your reactions may stem from childhood; if you have been bullied at school or have been made to feel inadequate in some way, this may be a factor and a reason why you may be quick to rise to anger or become defensive. Conflict is not necessarily to be avoided at all costs; conflict can be energising and will clear the air when managed effectively. However, when there is a hidden power dynamic at play, a more sinister aspect of workplace behaviour may arise. The next section will shed light on the dark side of conflict in the workplace; learning to recognise the signs of bullying can also help you to prevent and deal with more challenging conflict situations.

# Bullying at work

As you begin your final year, you will become conscious that you will soon be managing other colleagues. A key aspect of your responsibilities as a manager will be to ensure that staff are properly supported, and you will need to learn to recognise and help staff to report uncivil or bullying behaviour.

The NHS is fundamentally a caring organisation but has not always dealt with bullying effectively. However, over the last decade, bullying in the NHS has become a much more widely researched topic, and there have been some positive outcomes from new interventions. The British Medical Association (BMA) has mainly driven improvements, but the Royal College of Nursing (RCN) and other unions are also sources of guidance and support.

### Research summary: Bullying and harassment

Research has shown that 20 per cent of NHS staff reported being bullied at work and 43 per cent have witnessed bullying. NHS staff survey data (West et al., 2012) as well

*(Continued)*

(Continued)

as a report from the Race Equality Foundation (Kline, 2015) show that staff from a black and ethnic minority background are more likely than white staff to experience harassment, bullying or abuse from other staff. Bullying is a persistent problem in healthcare organisations and has significant negative outcomes for individuals and organisations (Carter et al., 2013). Following a review of policy and evidence, a recent BMA report makes recommendations for improvement to 'change the culture in the NHS and profession so that everyone is treated with respect and compassion' (BMA, 2018).

Activity 11.6 is designed to help you recognise the signs and to tackle bullying as you progress in your career and start thinking of yourself as a leader.

## Activity 11.6   Decision-making

**Part 1**

Think of an experience at work where you witnessed rude or disrespectful staff behaviour that made you feel uncomfortable.

What did you do? On reflection, is there anything else you could have done?

*As Part 1 of this activity is based on your own observation, there is no outline answer at the end of the chapter.*

**Part 2**

1.   What are some examples of bullying or uncivil behaviour at work?
2.   What are the signs of someone being bullied at work?
3.   What would you do if you suspected that a colleague was being bullied at work?

*An outline answer to Part 2 of this activity is given at the end of the chapter.*

As future managers and leaders in the NHS, student nurses have a responsibility to learn to speak up when things go wrong and to advocate for patients under their care. Speaking up demands great courage, and you will need to develop the confidence to trust in your own beliefs and values. The next section aims to give you the knowledge and confidence to voice your opinion in the most positive and effective way.

# Assertive communication

Although they may seem quite similar in meaning, there is a distinct difference between aggressive behaviour and assertive behaviour. On a scale of 0–10, passive behaviour is at one end of the scale (0) and aggressive behaviour is at the other (10); assertiveness lies somewhere close to the middle.

A *passive* communication is where the individual's needs, wishes, desires or concerns are not expressed explicitly. An *aggressive* communication involves pushing or forcing one's needs, wishes, desires or concerns on to another person.

In *assertive* communication, there are clearly two participants; two people may equally express their needs, and both have opportunities to listen and respond to one another without defensiveness (Raskin, 2013, p187).

An assertive message is an open one that facilitates or enhances effective communication, understanding and/or closure. Your non-verbal communication should always align with your spoken communication (for more detail, see Raskin, 2013). Activity 11.7 will help you to identify how assertive you are.

## Activity 11.7   Communication

Complete the 'How Assertive Am I?' quiz listed in the useful websites at the end of this chapter.

If the results indicate that you are lacking in assertiveness, formulate an action plan to identify learning objectives to help you become more assertive.

*As this activity is unique to you, there is no outline answer at the end of the chapter.*

Start setting yourself the learning and development objectives you have identified during the course of this chapter and focus on identifying and achieving your goal. The sky is the limit once you overcome any self-limiting beliefs, and the next section is designed to help you obtain the perfect first job.

# Preparing for employment

Once you begin your final year as a student nurse, you should start to think about the jobs and opportunities that will be available to you once you have qualified. Some students will have a clear picture of the career path they wish to take, but don't worry if you don't. You may not be able to decide yet, or you may have already realised that you are interested in specialising in one area. Many student nurses have childcare or other caring responsibilities, so look for a job that will offer flexible working or family-friendly shift patterns. If you are undecided, you can look for job opportunities across different settings such as hospitals, nursing homes, community nursing, armed forces, the private sector and hospices.

Your first job is a stepping stone towards the rest of your career; choose well and your first role will offer you the support you need to develop your confidence, consolidate your learning, and develop new skills and knowledge.

# First steps: the interview

In most cases, you will be likely to have a traditional interview and will be interviewed by two or more members of a selection panel.

You may come across other forms of interview, such as:

- assessment centre – these can last up to a day and have a number of components, such as group exercises, role plays, presentation, psychometrics and in-tray exercises;
- telephone or video conference;
- interview panel with two or more interviewers; and
- stress interview – designed to test your ability to think on your feet.

Beware of the informal interview that might happen if they decide to show you around the site. The interviewer may be trying to see what you are like when you are off guard. Stay alert and show interest, as well as asking appropriate questions.

# Preparation for interview: secret to success

The secret to success in interviews is preparation and practice; when you go for an interview, you should leave nothing to chance. Preparation can be divided into four categories:

1. Practical preparation:
   - Read the interview letter carefully; make sure you know who will interview you, what the format will be and how long it will take.
   - Do a trial run to make sure you know exactly how long to allow for the journey; check parking and public transport information.
   - Show enthusiasm and interest in the job – telephone to confirm your attendance.
   - If you have been asked to give a presentation, follow the brief exactly. Practice makes perfect, so rehearse out loud and stick to the time limit.
2. Research the organisation:
   - You may well have done your research but being knowledgeable about the organisation always impresses employers because it shows you are genuinely interested. You would be surprised at how many candidates don't do this.

- Be familiar with key things such as the philosophy of the organisation, numbers of staff and financial reporting.
- You can get this information from the organisation website, Care Quality Commission reports, open minutes from board meetings, financial reports, and staff survey results. Don't be shy about asking the employer for material in advance.

3. Match yourself to the role:

- Read the job description and person specification thoroughly.
- If this information has not been provided, ask the organisation to send it to you.
- If you are not entirely certain the job is right for you, ask if you can arrange an informal visit.
- Update your CV; read through the application form to remind yourself what you have written. Make sure your skills and achievements match the requirements.

4. Predict likely questions:

- The questions will depend on the format of the interview.
- In order to perform well, anticipate the questions you are most likely to get; prepare and practice your answers out loud in front of a family member or friend. This will help you to overcome your nerves. In the event that you have a momentary 'brain freeze', it is perfectly acceptable to ask the interviewer to repeat the question or if you can have some more time or return to the question later. Interviewers will expect candidates to display some nerves. Don't forget to prepare and practise some questions to ask the employer (e.g. what does their preceptorship programme look like?).

## Types of interview questions

You will be asked a range of questions at interview. Most will fall under the following categories:

- open;
- closed;
- hypothetical ('what if ...?');
- scenarios;
- leading;
- probing; and
- multiple-choice.

Some typical interview questions are listed in Table 11.3. Use this table to undertake Activity 11.8.

| |
|---|
| a) At times the nursing environment can be stressful. How do you manage stressful situations? |
| b) Give me an example of one of your strengths and an area of weakness. |
| c) What do think the role of a Band 5 nurse entails? |
| d) How do you ensure you keep up to date with current practices? |
| e) Why do you think we should give you this job? |
| f) How would you manage if you had a disagreement with a colleague about a patient's care? |
| g) What would you do if a patient's relative became angry with you? |

*Table 11.3*   Typical interview questions

## Activity 11.8   Communication

Prepare your answers, remembering to mention what you do well; practise your answers out loud. Ask a friend or family member to interview you using these questions.

*As this activity is based on your own observation, there is no outline answer at the end of the chapter.*

# The interview itself

## Personal presentation

As you know, first impressions count more than they probably should, so take time on the day to get this right. Most interviewers will be dressed conservatively, so make sure that you do the same. Dress appropriately for the job you are going for; you also need to make sure you appear relaxed and confident, so dress should be comfortable – not too tight or restrictive. Obviously, good personal hygiene is essential; don't smoke or drink immediately before the interview and make sure your shoes are clean and polished. Keep jewellery to a minimum and avoid strong perfumes (or aftershave) and brightly coloured scarves or ties. Take a document case with you to neatly store any papers you may need (e.g. supporting documents, notes, any questions you may want to ask them).

Make sure that you have a warm drink and snack about an hour beforehand to maintain your energy levels and take some water with you in case of delays.

## When you arrive

Aim to get there about ten minutes early. If you feel nervous, try breathing deeply, smile and be friendly with reception staff, and remember the key selling points you want to get across.

## The beginning of the interview

Greet the interviewer(s) confidently, maintain eye contact, smile and shake their hand firmly. Sit well back in your seat when you are asked to sit down, and keep your hands loosely in your lap – don't fidget, click or tap pens, and try to control any shaking arms or legs. Be aware of the interviewer's body language and your own, but don't let this interfere with your natural style.

## During the interview

Show interest and attention; try to speak a little more slowly than normal and keep a natural conversational tone. Make sure you get your key messages across and steer them to ask questions that will enable you to show your main skills and achievements. Don't worry about silence; take thinking time if you need it – don't waffle or lie, and keep your answers concise and to the point.

## The end of the interview

Ensure that you take the opportunity to ask your prepared questions; try to close on a positive note, which confirms to the interviewer that you are right for the job. Never discuss salary unless the interviewer raises it or they make you a definite offer at the time. Thank the interviewer at the end, shake hands and restate your interest in the job.

Once it's over, do something to unwind (e.g. meet a friend, go for a coffee or a walk). While it is fresh in your mind, reflect on how you performed; make a note of what you struggled with and what went well.

## Follow-up

If appropriate, email to thank the interviewer for their time; send any documents they asked for or you promised. If you don't hear back within the time frame they gave you, contact them; it shows genuine interest – not hearing does not always mean that you have failed. No matter the outcome of the interview, ask them for feedback; all interviews are a learning opportunity, whether you are successful or not.

Within your first job, it is likely that you will receive support to help with your transition from student to registered nurse through a preceptorship programme.

# Preceptorship

The Department of Health (2010) defines preceptorship as:

> *A period of structured transition for the newly registered practitioner during which he or she will be supported by a preceptor, to develop their confidence as an autonomous professional, refine skills, values and behaviours and to continue on their journey of life-long learning.*

(p11)

Preceptorship should be available to all newly registered nurses, but it is up to each organisation to decide who can access preceptorship, and hence programmes may vary. The overall aim of a preceptorship programme is to develop competent and confident practitioners, but preceptorship may be used by other professional groups such as overseas nurses, return to practice nurses, or new to general practice nurses, and is also relevant for allied health professionals.

Research indicates that many newly qualified nurses leave the profession if they do not receive the right support early in their career, so before you go for that first job interview, look at the RCN guidance to make sure you understand what should be offered by a preceptorship programme; look at what is on offer nationally and in other organisations so that you are equipped to negotiate the best terms of employment. Make sure that you receive the best support possible in your first year as a newly qualified nurse; follow the recommendations in this book and seek support from your university lecturers and partners in the practice area to ensure that you have an enjoyable, successful and long career in nursing.

---

### Chapter summary

This chapter has looked at some practical ways for you to develop some of the main skills and attributes you will need to equip you for your first job and the considerable responsibility of becoming a qualified nurse. Nursing is a profession unlike any other; we are privileged to be able to advocate for patients and be responsible for upholding their safety. Sometimes this can present quite a challenge, so you will need to muster your best qualities to set an example for others, and you will learn not to be intimidated by those who are senior to you when the need arises. We discussed that the first step towards development of your leadership is to become more self-aware; learning to understand your own behaviour will help you to understand others, and as you develop confidence you will get the best out of yourself and other team members. It is also essential to reflect and learn from your mistakes; set yourself development goals so that you will become a nurse who is proud of your profession and everything it stands for.

---

## Activities: brief outline answers

### Activity 11.1   Team working (p198)

1. The student nurse adopted the do-it-all style and began doing observations followed by other tasks without agreeing allocation of tasks with her team colleague, Sonya. This is an example of ineffective delegation leading to a breakdown in teamwork (Magnusson et al., 2017).

2. When you are working with an HCA or another member of staff, it is important to discuss and agree distribution of tasks so that each of you understands your responsibilities. Agreeing how to share the workload will also help to build a positive, supportive working

relationship so that when emergencies occur you will be able to work effectively as a team. Offers of support are much more likely to be reciprocated if instructions are clear and communication channels kept friendly, confident and open.

## Activity 11.6    Decision-making (p206)

1.    What are some examples of bullying or uncivil behaviour at work?

- Having your views and opinions ignored.
- Being humiliated or ridiculed in connection with your work.
- Being shouted at or being the target of spontaneous anger.
- Spreading gossip or rumours about individual work colleagues.
- Being reminded of your mistakes.
- Pressure not to claim something to which you are entitled (e.g. sick leave, holiday entitlement).
- Persistent criticism of your work and effort.
- Intimidating behaviour (finger-pointing, invasion of personal space, shoving or blocking the way).
- Threats of violence or physical abuse (or actual abuse).
- Being subjected to teasing or sarcasm.
- Insulting remarks about your person (habits, background) or your attitudes or private life.

2.    What are the signs of someone being bullied at work?

- Insomnia and inability to relax.
- Loss of confidence and self-doubt.
- Loss of appetite.
- Hypervigilance and excessive double-checking of all actions.
- Inability to switch off from work.

3.    What would you do if you suspected that a colleague was being bullied at work?

- If you are a student, follow the raising concerns policy and discuss with your university lecturer or personal tutor.
- If you are qualified, recognise your rights; make sure you/they are aware of organisational policy related to bullying and harassment at work.
- Seek advice and support from an RCN or union representative.
- Read the RCN guidance (RCN, 2019b).

## Further reading

**Kline, R.** (2015) *Beyond the Snowy White Peaks of the NHS?* Available at: http://raceequalityfoundation.org.uk/wp-content/uploads/2018/02/Health-Briefing-39-_Final.pdf

An important read for all nurses, identifying the problems that still exist for black minority ethnic staff in the NHS.

**NHS Improvement** (2018) *Managing Conflict.* Available at: https://improvement.nhs.uk/documents/2130/managing-conflict.pdf

A helpful resource with strategies to manage conflict at work.

**Royal College of Nursing (RCN)** (2017) *Accountability and Delegation.* Available at: www.rcn.org.uk/professional-development/accountability-and-delegation

A useful overview applicable to all members of the nursing team, including students.

**Royal College of Nursing (RCN)** (2019) *Bullying and Harassment.* Available at: www.rcn.org.uk/get-help/rcn-advice/bullying-and-harassment

This guide is a good resource if you or a colleague are experiencing bullying or harassment at work.

**Royal College of Nursing (RCN)** (2019) *NMC: Preceptorship.* Available at: www.rcn.org.uk/get-help/rcn-advice/nursing-and-midwifery-council-precept

This web page has a range of resources and guidance to help you prepare for preceptorship when you qualify.

## Useful websites

Assertiveness Quiz

**www.compasstoolkit.ox.ac.uk/wp-content/uploads/2015/11/Assertiveness-Quiz-Tips-Individual-Activity.pdf**

A quick quiz to identify how assertive you are.

Belbin's Team Roles

**www.belbin.com/media/1335/belbin-for-lecturers.pdf**

Team working is essential in nursing, and this provides a useful summary of the different roles people play in a team. Which one are you?

Conflict Style Questionnaire

**https://edge.sagepub.com/sites/default/files/10.2_Conflict_Style_Questionnaire.pdf**

A quick quiz to identify your conflict style.

Johari Window: Video Explanation

**www.youtube.com/watch?v=KdYo5jn29w4**

A presentation that explains how understanding yourself and others can be helpful in life and work relationships.

Just a Routine Operation

**www.youtube.com/watch?v=JzlvgtPIof4**

This video is useful to understand the importance of assertive communication; it also outlines principles of human factors.

# Glossary

**annual appraisal**   A structured meeting to provide feedback on performance and identify development needs.

**assistive technology**   Technology that can help people with their daily life (e.g. hearing aids, screen readers, educational software, memory aids).

**attention deficit hyperactivity disorder (ADHD)**   A behavioural disorder in which children and adults may have difficulty with inattentiveness or hyperactivity and impulsiveness.

**autistic spectrum disorder (ASD)**   The brain in people with ASD works in a different way to other people. They may find it difficult to communicate or interact with other people and understand how they think or feel. They can be upset by loud noises, bright lights or being in unfamiliar situations. It is not a medical condition, and individuals require support to manage certain areas of their life.

**British National Formulary (BNF)**   Available in print, online or as an app, it provides information about an extensive range of medicines, including uses, contraindications, side effects, dosages and costs.

**child and adolescent mental health services (CAMHS)**   A range of services for children and young people who have difficulties with emotional or behavioural well-being.

**clinical decision-making**   The application of clinical judgement to select the best evidence to inform effective clinical care.

**conflict management**   The use of techniques to minimise the negative effects of a conflict while maximising the positives.

**Disabled Students' Allowances (DSAs)**   Additional allowances available to students to assist them with the additional costs they may have due to their additional needs (e.g. specialist equipment to help them with their studies, to pay for costs of non-medical helpers, additional travel costs).

**Disclosure and Barring Service (DBS)**   Enables employers to check if a person has a criminal record (i.e. any spent and unspent convictions, cautions, reprimands and final warnings), as well as any information held by the police that is considered relevant to your role.

**dyscalculia**   A specific learning disability where an individual has difficulties with arithmetical skills.

**dyslexia**   A specific learning difficulty where an individual has difficulties with reading, writing and spelling.

**dyspraxia**   A specific learning difficulty where an individual has difficulty with spatial and perceptual skills.

**electronic patient records**   A number of different software applications that bring all of a patient's data together, which is now replacing paper records for patients.

**enuresis nurse specialist**   A nurse who specialises in working with children who suffer from involuntary urination (e.g. bed-wetting – nocturnal enuresis – by children over the age of 5 years).

**fitness to practise**   A term used by the NMC. Being fit to practise requires a nurse or midwife to have the skills, knowledge, good health and good character to do their job safely and effectively, and so be on the NMC register without restriction.

**induction booklet**   A booklet provided by many placements that provides details of the placement, learning opportunities available, keywords used and recommended reading.

**information governance and data security**   Relates to the secure storage and handling of personal data, and ensuring it is collected, stored, used and shared appropriately.

**integrated health and social care**   A government policy to develop better coordination between hospitals, the community and social care organisations in order to provide seamless care for people, particularly the elderly and those with long-term conditions.

**mental distress**   Problems with thinking or feeling that can impact on a person's ability to cope in day-to-day life, including fear, anxiety, depression, confusion and mood swings.

**mentors and sign-off mentors**   Terms to describe the registered nurses who supported students in practice. Mentors both supervised and assessed students. Sign-off mentors would confirm that a student had achieved the required proficiency to demonstrate safe and effective practice to enter the NMC register at the end of their programme. These roles have now been replaced by practice supervisors and assessors.

**National Institute for Health and Care Excellence (NICE)**   An organisation set up to produce authoritative national guidance on the use of new and existing technologies.

**objective, evidence-based assessment**   Reliable assessment by a practice assessor that is based on a range of evidence, such as student records, direct observations, student self-reflection and feedback from others (nurses and other health and social care professionals).

**Objective Structured Clinical Assessments or Examinations (OSCAs or OSCEs)**
Assessments of clinical competence carried out in a structured and objective way. They are commonly used in pre- and post-registration programmes. The format usually comprises of a number of assessment stations that students must rotate round, with various tasks/scenarios at each one.

**Ongoing Achievement Record (OAR)**   A document that summarises your achievement on each placement. It may be a separate document from your Practice Assessment Document or integrated into it.

**person-centred care**   An approach that puts people at the centre of care and involves collaborative working and shared decision-making.

**Practice Assessment Document (PAD)**   The document that students take out to practice (hard copy or electronic) which contains all the skills/proficiencies/learning outcomes that a student has to achieve in practice. Different HEIs may use different terms.

**practice partners**   A term commonly used to describe the organisations that offer placements to students and work with universities in supporting and developing the curriculum and the student experience.

**preceptorship**   A period of time when a newly qualified nurse is provided with support by a preceptor to make the transition to their new role. This can be anything from 6 to 12 months.

**professional socialisation**   Acquiring the skills, knowledge and values of a group; in the context of this book, it relates to the nursing profession.

**rota**   A record of all staff on a placement and the shifts they are working for a given time period.

**skills and simulation suites or laboratories**   Permanent or flexible facilities that replicate the different environments students will experience on placement (e.g. a ward, a GP practice, a person's home). They can be fully equipped with hospital beds and a range of clinical equipment found in different healthcare environments. They provide safe environments for students to acquire, develop and refine clinical skills in a safe and supportive environment.

**social psychology**   A scientific discipline that explores and explains how the thoughts, behaviours and feelings of an individual are shaped by the presence of others.

**therapeutic skills**   A range of communication and social skills that nurses use when engaging with patients (e.g. empathy, listening skills, use of silence, reflecting, paraphrasing, summarising) to develop a relationship based on mutual trust and respect.

# References

Ash, A. (2016) *Whistleblowing and Ethics in Health and Social Care*. London: Jessica Kingsley Publishers.

Asselin, M., Schwartz-Barcott, D. and Osterman, P. (2013) Exploring reflection as a process embedded in experienced nurses' practice: a qualitative study. *Journal of Advanced Nursing*, 69(4): 905–14.

Avis, M. and Freshwater, D. (2006) Evidence for practice, epistemology and critical reflection. *Nursing Philosophy*, 7(4): 216–24.

Benner, P. (1984) *From Novice to Expert*. Menlo Park, CA: Addison-Wesley.

Berwick, D. (2013) *A Promise to Learn – A Commitment to Act: Improving the Safety of Patients in England*. London: Department of Health.

Borrott, N., Day, G.E., Sedgwick, M. and Levett-Jones, T. (2016) Nursing students' belongingness and workplace satisfaction: quantitative findings of a mixed methods study. *Nurse Education Today*, 45: 29–34.

Borton, T. (1970) *Reach, Touch and Teach*. London: Hutchinson.

Brady, M., Price, J., Bolland, R. and Finnerty, G. (2017) Needing to belong: first practice placement experiences of children's nursing students. *Comprehensive Child and Adolescent Nursing*, 42(1): 24–39.

Bramley, L. and Matiti, M. (2014) How does it really feel to be in my shoes? Patients' compassion within nursing care and their perceptions of developing compassionate nurses. *Journal of Clinical Nursing*, 23(19–20): 2790–9.

Briscoe, L. (2013) Becoming culturally sensitive: a painful process? *Midwifery*, 29(6): 559–65.

Bristol Royal Infirmary Inquiry (2001) *Learning from Bristol: The Report of the Public Inquiry into Children's Heart Surgery at the Bristol Royal Infirmary 1984–1995*. Available at: https://webarchive.nationalarchives.gov.uk/20090811143822/http:/www.bristol-inquiry.org.uk/final_report/the_report.pdf

British Dyslexia Association (n.d.) *Dyslexia*. Available at: www.bdadyslexia.org.uk/dyslexia

British Medical Association (BMA) (2018) *Bullying and Harassment: How to Address It and Create a Supportive and Inclusive Culture*. London: BMA.

Brooker, C. and Waugh, A. (2013) *Foundations of Nursing Practice: Fundamentals of Holistic Care*, 2nd edn. London: Mosby.

Button, L., Green, B., Tengnah, C., Johansson, I. and Baker, C. (2005) The impact of international placements on nurses' personal and professional lives: literature review. *Journal of Advanced Nursing*, 50(3): 315–24.

Carper, B. (1978) Fundamental ways of knowing in nursing. *Advances in Nursing Science*, 1(1): 13–23.

Carter, M., Thompson, N., Crampton P., Morrow, G., Burford, B., Gray, G. and Illing, J. (2013) *Workplace Bullying in the UK NHS: A Questionnaire and Interview Study on Prevalence, Impact and Barriers to Reporting.* Available at: https://bmjopen.bmj.com/content/bmjopen/3/6/e002628.full.pdf

Cavendish, C. (2013) *Cavendish Review: An Independent Enquiry into Healthcare Assistants and Support Workers in the NHS and Social Care Setting.* Available at: www.gov.uk/government/publications/review-of-healthcare-assistants-and-support-workers-in-nhs-and-social-care

Cope, V. and Murray, M. (2018) Use of professional portfolios in nursing. *Nursing Standard*, 32(50): 55–63.

Council of Deans of Health (CoDH) (2016) *Supporting Nursing, Midwifery and Allied Health Professional Students to Raise Concerns with the Quality of Care.* Available at: https://councilofdeans.org.uk/

Department of Health (2010) *Preceptorship Framework for Newly Registered Nurses, Midwives and Allied Health Professionals.* Available at: https://webarchive.nationalarchives.gov.uk/20130105024308/http://www.dh.gov.uk/prod_consum_dh/groups/dh_digitalassets/@dh/@en/@abous/documents/digitalasset/dh_114116.pdf

Department of Health (2012) *Transforming Care: A National Response to Winterbourne View Hospital Department of Health Review – Final Report.* Available at: www.gov.uk/government/publications/winterbourne-view-hospital-department-of-health-review-and-response

Department of Health and NHS Commissioning Board (2012) *Compassion in Practice: Nursing, Midwifery and Care Staff – Our Vision and Strategy.* Available at: www.england.nhs.uk/wp-content/uploads/2012/12/compassion-in-practice.pdf

Dewey, J. (1933) *How We Think: A Reinstatement of the Reation of Reflective Thinking to the Education Process.* Boston, MA: D.C. Heath.

Doody, O., Tuohy, D. and Deasy, C. (2012) Final-year student nurses' perceptions of role transition. *British Journal of Nursing*, 21(11): 684–8.

Duffy, K. (2003) *Failing Students: A Qualitative Study of Factors that Influence the Decisions Regarding Assessment of Students' Competence in Practice.* Available at: https://tinyurl.com/yca7t4vu

Duffy, K. (2006) *Weighing the Balance.* PhD thesis, Glasgow Caledonian University.

Duffy, K. (2013) Providing constructive feedback to students during mentoring. *Nursing Standard*, 27(31): 50–6.

Duffy, M.E., Farmer, S., Ravert, P. and Huittinen, L. (2005) International community health networking project: two-year follow-up of graduates. *International Nursing Review*, 52(1): 24–31.

Dunbar, H. and Carter, B. (2017) A sense of belonging: the importance of fostering student nurses' affective bonds. *Journal of Child Health Care*, 21(4): 367–9.

Elcock, K. (2013) Raising concerns in an open culture. *British Journal of Nursing*, 22(19): 1140.

Equality and Human Rights Commission (EHRC) (2019) *What Are Reasonable Adjustments? When Is It Reasonable for a Further or Higher Education Institution to Make Adjustments?* Available at: www.equalityhumanrights.com/en/advice-and-guidance/what-are-reasonable-adjustments

Flynn, M. (2012) *Winterbourne View Hospital: A Serious Case Review*. Available at: https://hosted.southglos.gov.uk/wv/report.pdf

Fowler, J. (2014) Reflection: from staff nurse to nurse consultant. *British Journal of Nursing*, 23(3): 176.

Francis, R. (2010) *The Independent Inquiry into Care Provided by Mid Staffordshire NHS Foundation Trust, January 2005–March 2009*. London: The Stationery Office.

Francis, R. (2013) *Report of the Mid Staffordshire NHS Foundation Trust Public Inquiry*. Available at: www.gov.uk/government/publications/report-of-the-mid-staffordshire-nhs-foundation-trust-public-inquiry

Francis, R. (2015) *Freedom to Speak Up: An Independent Review into Creating an Open and Honest Reporting Culture in the NHS*. Available at: http://freedomtospeakup.org.uk/the-report/

Freudenberger, H.J. (1974) Staff burnout. *Journal of Social Issues*, 30(1): 159–65.

Gallagher, R. (2013) Compassion fatigue. *Canadian Family Physician*, 59(3): 265–8.

Gault, I., Shapcott, J., Luthi, A. and Reid, G. (2017) *Communication in Nursing and Healthcare*. London: SAGE.

Gibbs, G. (1988) *Learning by Doing: A Guide to Teaching and Learning Methods*. Oxford: Further Education Unit, Oxford Polytechnic.

Gillespie, M. and Rivers, I. (2017) Assistant grade nurses and nursing students: a diary study. *Mental Health Practice*, 21(3): 21–5.

Goleman, D. (1999) *Working with Emotional Intelligence*. London: Bloomsbury Publishing.

Gosport Independent Panel (2018) *Gosport War Memorial Hospital: The Report of the Gosport Independent Panel*. Available at: www.gosportpanel.independent.gov.uk

Green, J., Jester, R., McKinley, R. and Pooler, A. (2014) The impact of chronic venous leg ulcers: a systematic review. *Journal of Wound Care*, 23(12): 601–12.

Hasson, F., McKenna, H.P. and Keeney, S. (2013) Perceptions of the unregistered healthcare worker's role in pre-registration student nurses' clinical training. *Journal of Advanced Nursing*, 69(7): 1618–29.

Health and Safety Executive (HSE) (2018) *Health and Safety at Work: Summary Statistics for Great Britain 2018*. Available at: www.hse.gov.uk/Statistics/overall/hssh1718.pdf

Health Education England (HEE) (2015) *Raising the Bar: Shape of Caring – A Review of the Future Education and Training of Registered Nurses and Care Assistants*. Available at: www.hee.nhs.uk/sites/default/files/documents/2348-Shape-of-caring-review-FINAL.pdf

Health Education England (HEE) (2018) *Maximising Leadership Learning in the Pre-Registration Healthcare Curricula.* Available at: www.hee.nhs.uk/sites/default/files/documents/Guidelines%20-%20Maximising%20Leadership%20in%20the%20Pre-reg%20Healthcare%20Curricula%20%282018%29.pdf

Higher Education Statistics Agency (HESA) (2019) *Undergraduate Declared Disabilities, UK Higher Education Sector, Nursing Students (JACS Code B7), 2012–2017.* Cheltenham: HESA.

Hunt, L.A., McGee, P., Gutteridge, R. and Hughes, M. (2012) Assessment of student nurses in practice: a comparison of theoretical and practical assessment results in England. *Nurse Education Today,* 32(4): 351–5.

Hunt, L.A., McGee, P., Gutteridge, R. and Hughes, M. (2014) Failing securely: the processes and support which underpin English nurse mentors' assessment decisions regarding under-performing students. *Nurse Education Today,* 39: 79–86.

Infection Control Team (2016) *Standard Infection Control Precautions (SICPs) Literature Review: Hand Hygiene – Hand Washing in the Hospital Setting.* Available at: www.nipcm.hps.scot.nhs.uk/documents/sicp-hand-hygiene-hand-washing-in-the-hospital-setting/

Ion, R., Jones, A. and Craven, R. (2016) Raising concerns and reporting poor care in practice. *Nursing Standard,* 31(15): 55–61.

Jackson, D., Firtko, A. and Edenborough, M. (2007) Personal resilience as a strategy for surviving and thriving in the face of workplace adversity: a literature review. *Journal of Advanced Nursing,* 60(1): 1–9.

Jackson, D., Hutchinson, M., Bronwyn, E., Mannix, J., Peters, K. and Weaver, R. (2011) Struggling for legitimacy: nursing students' stories of organisational aggression, resilience and resistance. *Nursing Inquiry,* 18(2): 102–10.

Johns, C. (1995) Framing learning through reflection within Carper's fundamental ways of knowing in nursing. *Journal of Advanced Nursing,* 22(2): 226–34.

Jones, L. and Bennett, C. (2012) *Leadership in Health and Social Care: An Introduction for Emerging Leaders.* Banbury: Lantern Publishing.

Keogh, B. (2013) *Review into the Quality of Care and Treatment Provided by 14 Hospital Trusts in England: Overview Report.* London: NHS England.

Kirkup, B. (2015) *The Report of the Morecambe Bay Investigation.* Available at: https://assets.publishing.service.gov.uk/government/uploads/system/uploads/attachment_data/file/408480/47487_MBI_Accessible_v0.1.pdf

Kline, R. (2015) *Beyond the Snowy White Peaks of the NHS?* Available at: http://raceequalityfoundation.org.uk/wp-content/uploads/2018/02/Health-Briefing-39-_Final.pdf

Lankshear, A. (1990) Failing to fail: the teacher's dilemma. *Nursing Standard,* 4(20): 35–7.

Lengelle, R., Luken, T. and Meijers, F. (2016) Is self-reflection dangerous? Preventing rumination in career learning. *Australian Journal of Career Development,* 25(3): 99–199.

Lewis, T. (2012) *Proving Disability and Reasonable Adjustments: A Worker's Guide to Evidence under the Equality Act 2010,* 4th edn. London: Central London Law Centre.

MacDonald, K., Paterson, K., and Wallar, J. (2016) Nursing students' experience of practice placements. *Nursing Standard*, 31(10): 44–50.

Maginnis, C. (2018) A discussion of professional identity development in nursing students. *Journal of Perspectives in Applied Academic Practice*, 6(1): 91–7.

Magnusson, C., Allan, H., Horton, K., Jones, M., Evans, K. and Ball, E. (2017) An analysis of delegation styles among newly qualified nurses. *Nursing Standard*, 31(25): 46–53.

Maheady, D. (2006) *Leave No Nurse Behind: Nurses Working with Disabilities*. New York: iUniverse.

Marks, B. (2007) Cultural competence revisited: nursing students with disabilities. *Journal of Nursing Education*, 46(2): 70–4.

McClimens, A. and Brewster, J. (2017) Using the hub and spoke student placement model in learning disability settings. *Learning Disability Practice*, 20(3): 34–8.

McMahon-Parkes, K., Chapmain, L. and James, J. (2016) The views of patients, mentors and adult field nursing students on patients' participation in student nurse assessment in practice. *Nurse Education in Practice*, 16(1): 202–8.

McManus, S., Bebbington, P., Jenkins, R. and Brugha, T. (eds) (2016) *Mental Health and Wellbeing in England: Adult Psychiatric Morbidity Survey 2014*. Leeds: NHS Digital.

Meetoo, D. (2010) International electives: nursing idealism, or safaris? *British Journal of Nursing*, 19(11): 681.

Mental Health Foundation (2019) *Stress: Are We Coping?* Available at: www.mentalhealth.org.uk/a-to-z/s/stress

Middleton, J. (2017) *Excellence in Student Nursing Placements*. Available at: www.nhsemployers.org/your-workforce/plan/nursing-workforce/nursing-education-and-training/excellence-in-student-nursing-placements

Middleton, R. (2017) Is reflection 'overdone' in nursing education? *Australian Nursing and Midwifery Journal*, 25(2): 36.

Morgan, D. (2011) Student nurse perception of risk in relation to international placements: a phenomenological research study. *Nurse Education Today*, 32(8): 956–60.

Morris, H. (2014) *Metacognition: Cultivating Reflection to Help Students Become Self-Directed Learners*. Available at: https://lsa.umich.edu/content/dam/sweetland-assets/sweetland-documents/teachingresources/CultivatingReflectionandMetacognition/Metacognition.pdf

Neuberger, J.C. and Aaronovitch, D. (2013) *More Care, Less Pathway: A Review of the Liverpool Care Pathway*. London: Department of Health.

NHS (2018a) *Moodzone: 5 Steps to Mental Wellbeing*. Available at: www.nhs.uk/conditions/stress-anxiety-depression/improve-mental-wellbeing/

NHS (2018b) *Moodzone: Breathing Exercises for Stress*. Available at: www.nhs.uk/conditions/stress-anxiety-depression/ways-relieve-stress/

NHS (2018c) *Moodzone: Get Active for Mental Welbeing*. Available at: www.nhs.uk/conditions/stress-anxiety-depression/mental-benefits-of-exercise/

NHS (2019a) *Moodzone: Understanding Stress.* Available at: www.nhs.uk/conditions/stress-anxiety-depression/understanding-stress/

NHS (2019b) *The NHS Long Term Plan.* Available at: www.longtermplan.nhs.uk

NHS Improvement (2016) *Freedom to Speak Up: Raising Concerns (Whistleblowing) Policy for the NHS.* Available at: https://improvement.nhs.uk/documents/27/whistleblowing_policy_final.pdf

NHS Improvement (2018) *Managing Conflict.* Available at: https://improvement.nhs.uk/documents/2130/managing-conflict.pdf

Norton, D. and Marks-Maran, D. (2014) Developing cultural sensitivity and awareness in nursing overseas. *Nursing Standard,* 28(44): 39–43.

Nursing and Midwifery Council (NMC) (2017a) *Guidance on Using Social Media Responsibly.* Available at: www.nmc.org.uk/standards/guidance/social-media-guidance

Nursing and Midwifery Council (NMC) (2017b) *Annual Fitness to Practise Report 2016–2017.* Available at: www.nmc.org.uk/about-us/reports-and-accounts/fitness-to-practise-annual-report/

Nursing and Midwifery Council (NMC) (2017c) *Enabling Professionalism in Nursing and Midwifery Practice.* Available at: www.nmc.org.uk/globalassets/sitedocuments/other-publications/enabling-professionalism.pdf

Nursing and Midwifery Council (NMC) (2018a) *The Code: Professional Standards of Practice and Behaviour for Nurses, Midwives and Nursing Associates.* Available at: www.nmc.org.uk/standards/code/

Nursing and Midwifery Council (NMC) (2018b) *Realising Professionalism: Standards for Education and Training. Part 1: Standards Framework for Nursing and Midwifery Education.* Available at: www.nmc.org.uk/standards/standards-for-nurses/

Nursing and Midwifery Council (NMC) (2018c) *Realising Professionalism: Standards for Education and Training. Part 2: Standards for Student Supervision and Assessment.* Available at: www.nmc.org.uk/standards/standards-for-nurses/

Nursing and Midwifery Council (NMC) (2018d) *Realising Professionalism: Standards for Education and Training. Part 3: Standards for Pre-Registration Nursing Programmes.* Available at: www.nmc.org.uk/standards/standards-for-nurses/

Nursing and Midwifery Council (NMC) (2018e) *Future Nurse: Standards of Proficiency for Registered Nurses.* Available at: www.nmc.org.uk/standards/standards-for-nurses/

Nursing and Midwifery Council (NMC) (2018f) *Raising Concerns: Guidance for Nurses, Midwives and Nursing Associates.* Available at: www.nmc.org.uk/globalassets/blocks/media-block/raising-concerns-v2.pdf

Nursing and Midwifery Council (NMC) (2018g) *Delegation and Accountability: Supplementary Information to the NMC Code.* Available at: www.nmc.org.uk/globalassets/sitedocuments/nmc-publications/delegation-and-accountability-supplementary-information-to-the-nmc-code.pdf

Nursing and Midwifery Council (NMC) (2019) *Revalidation.* Available at: www.nmc.org.uk/globalassets/sitedocuments/revalidation/how-to-revalidate-booklet.pdf

Office for Disability Issues (2011) *Equality Act 2010 Guidance: Guidance on Matters to Be Taken into Account in Determining Questions Relating to the Definition of Disability.* Available at: https://assets.publishing.service.gov.uk/government/uploads/system/uploads/attachment_data/file/570382/Equality_Act_2010-disability_definition.pdf

Open University (2006) *Making Your Teaching Inclusive.* Available at: www.open.ac.uk/inclusiveteaching

Pan London Practice Learning Group (PLPLG) (2019) *The Pan London Practice Assessment Document (PLPAD 2.0).* Available at: https://plplg.uk

Peña-Sarrionandia, A., Mikolajcak, M. and Gross, J. (2015) Integrating emotional regulation and emotional intelligence traditions: a meta analysis. *Frontiers in Psychology,* 6(160). doi: 10.3389/fpsyg.2015.00160

Pollack, D. (2009) *Neurodiversity in Higher Education: Positive Responses to Specific Learning Differences.* Chichester: Wiley-Blackwell.

Price, A. (2004) Encouraging reflection and critical thinking in practice. *Nursing Standard,* 18(7): 46–52.

Raskin, P.M. (2013) Confident communication. In E.L.M. Rigolosi (ed), *Management and Leadership in Nursing and Healthcare: An Experiential Approach,* 3rd edn. New York: Springer, pp179–200.

Quappe, S. and Cantatore, G. (2005) *What Is Cultural Awareness Anyway? How Do I Build It?* Available at: www.culturosity.com/pdfs/What%20is%20Cultural%20Awareness.pdf

Reed, S. (2015) *Successful Professional Portfolios for Nursing Students.* Exeter: Learning Matters.

Rolfe, G., Freshwater, J. and Jasper, M. (2001) *Critical Reflection in Nursing and the Helping Professions: A User's Guide.* Basingstoke: Palgrave Macmillan.

Royal College of Nursing (RCN) (2017a) *Helping Students Get the Best from Their Practice Placements: A Royal College of Nursing Toolkit.* Available at: www.rcn.org.uk/professional-development/publications/pub-006035

Royal College of Nursing (RCN) (2017b) *RCN Guidance for Mentors of Nursing and Midwifery Students.* London: RCN.

Royal College of Nursing (RCN) (2018a) *Training: Statutory and Mandatory.* Available at: www.rcn.org.uk/get-help/rcn-advice/training-statutory-and-mandatory

Royal College of Nursing (RCN) (2018b) *Student Electives Overseas: Advice Guides.* Available at: www.rcn.org.uk/get-help/rcn-advice/student-electives-overseas

Royal College of Nursing (RCN) (2019a) *Statements: How to Write Them.* Available at: www.rcn.org.uk/get-help/rcn-advice/statements

Royal College of Nursing (RCN) (2019b) *Bullying and Harassment.* Available at: www.rcn.org.uk/get-help/rcn-advice/bullying-and-harassment

Rylance, R., Barrett, J., Sixsmith, P. and Ward, D. (2017) Student nurse mentoring: an evaluative study of the mentor's perspective. *British Journal of Nursing,* 26(7): 405–9.

Salman, S. (2018) Seven years on from Winterbourne View, why has nothing changed? *The Guardian*, 30 May. Available at: www.theguardian.com/society/2018/may/30/seven-years-winterbourne-view-learning-disabled-people-abuse

Salomon, G. and Perkins, D.(1989) Rocky roads to transfer: rethinking mechanisms of a neglected phenomenon. *Educational Psychologist*, 24(2): 113–42.

Save the Student (2019) *Student Living Costs in the UK 2019*. Available at: www.savethestudent.org/money/student-budgeting

Schon, D. (1983) *The Reflective Practitioner*. San Francisco, CA: Jossey-Bass.

Sharples, K. (2011) *Successful Practice Learning for Nursing Students*, 2nd edn. Exeter: Learning Matters.

Sharples, K. and Elcock, K. (2011) *Preceptorship for Newly Registered Nurses*. Exeter: Learning Matters.

Shepherd, P. and Uren, C. (2014) Protecting students' supernumerary status. *Nursing Times*, 10(20): 18–20.

Speers, J. and Lathlean, J. (2015) Service user involvement in giving mental health students feedback on placement: a participatory action research study. *Nurse Education Today*, 35(9): e84–e89.

Standage, R. and Randall, D. (2014) The benefits for children's nurses of overseas placements: where is the evidence? *Issues in Comprehensive Paediatric Nursing*, 37(20): 87–102.

Stanley, N., Ridley, J., Manthorpe, J., Harris, J. and Hurst, A. (2007) *Disclosing Disability: Disabled Students and Practitioners in Social Work, Nursing and Teaching*. London: Disability Rights Commission.

Sumner, J. (2010) Reflection and moral maturity in a nurse's caring practice. *Nursing Philosphy*, 11(3): 159–69.

Sung, K. (2006) Literature review on self-regulated learning. *Singapore Nursing Journal*, 33(2): 38–45.

Taylor, B., Roberts, S., Smyth, T. and Tulloch, M. (2015) Nurse managers' strategies for feeling less drained by their work: an action research and reflection project for developing emotional intelligence. *Journal of Nursing Management*, 23(7): 879–87.

Taylor, R. (2019) Contemporary issues: resilience training alone is an incomplete intervention. *Nurse Education Today*, 78: 10–13.

Taylor, R. and Fontaine, N. (2019) Leadership and management in nursing adults. In K. Elcock, W. Wright, P. Newcombe and F. Everett (eds), *Essentials of Nursing Adults*. London: SAGE, pp690–704.

Thomas, K.W. and Kilmann, R.H. (1974) *Thomas–Kilmann Conflict Mode Instrument*. Tuxedo, NY: Xicom.

Thomas, L. and Asselin, M. (2018) Promoting resilience among nursing students in clinical education. *Nurse Education in Practice*, 28: 231–4.

Thomas, M. and Westwood, N. (2016) Student experience of hub and spoke model of placement allocation: an evaluative study. *Nurse Education Today*, 46: 24–8.

Van Woerkom, M. (2010) Critical reflection as a rationalistic ideal. *Adult Education Quarterly*, 60(4): 339–56.

Werenberg, M. (2016) *Rumination: A Problem in Anxiety and Depression.* Available at: www.psychologytoday.com/au/blog/depression-management-techniques/201604/rumination-problem-in-anxiety-and-depression

West, M., Dawson, J., Admasachew, L. and Topakas, A. (2012) *NHS Staff Management and Health Service Quality: Results from the NHS Staff Survey and Related Data.* Available at: www.gov.uk/government/uploads/system/uploads/attachment_data/file/215455/dh_129656.pdf

Whitehead, B. (2013) Getting the most out of your clinical placement. *Nursing Times*, 109(37): 12–13.

World Health Organization (WHO) (2016) *Global Strategic Directions for Strengthening Nursing and Midwifery 2016–2020.* Paris: WHO Library.

World Health Organization (WHO) (2018) *International Statistical Classification of Diseases and Related Health Problems.* Available at: https://icd.who.int/browse11/l-m/en

YouGov (2016) *One in Four Students Suffer from Mental Health Problems.* Available at: yougov.co.uk/news/2016/08/09/quarter-britains-students-are-afflicted-mentalhea/

# Index